Fungal Infections of the Nail and Scalp

This new edition of a bestselling text has been expanded to include scalp infections; as before, this illustrated text has been written by clinicians for clinicians, to provide an authoritative guide to the steps needed to identify and effectively manage the patient with fungal nail or scalp infection.

T0321390

Fungal Infections of the Nail and Scalp

The Current Approach to Diagnosis and Therapy

Third Edition

Edited by

Robert Baran, MD

Honorary Professor, University of Franche-Comté;
Nail Disease Center, Cannes, France

Eckart Haneke, MD

Dermatology Practice, Dermaticum, Freiburg, Germany; Centro de Dermatología Epidermis, Instituto CUF, Porto, Portugal; Kliniek voor Huidziekten, Universitair Ziekenhuis, Ghent, Belgium; Department of Dermatology, Inselspital, University of Bern, Bern, Switzerland

Roderick Hay, DM, FMedSci

Emeritus Professor of Cutaneous Infection, Kings College London, and of Dermatology, Queens University Belfast; Consultant Dermatologist, London Bridge Hospital, UK

Antonella Tosti, MD

Fredric Brandt Endowed Professor of Dermatology, Dr. Phillip Frost Department of Dermatology and Cutaneous Surgery, University of Miami Miller School of Medicine, Miami, Florida, USA

Bertrand Richert-Baran, MD, PhD

Professor of Dermatology, Head and Chair, Brugmann & Saint Pierre University Hospitals, Université Libre de Bruxelles, Belgium

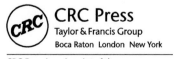

CRC Press
Taylor & Francis Group
Boca Raton London New York

CRC Press is an imprint of the
Taylor & Francis Group, an **informa** business

Designed cover image: Editors

Third edition published 2025
by CRC Press
2385 NW Executive Center Drive, Suite 320, Boca Raton FL 33431

and by CRC Press
4 Park Square, Milton Park, Abingdon, Oxon, OX14 4RN

CRC Press is an imprint of Taylor & Francis Group, LLC

ISBN: 9781032464329 (hbk)
ISBN: 9781032464305 (pbk)
ISBN: 9781003381648 (ebk)

DOI: 10.1201/9781003381648

Typeset in Palatino
by codeMantra

Contents

Contributors

Roberto Arenas
Hospital General "Dr. Manuel Gea
 González"
Mexico City, Mexico

Giuseppe Argenziano
Department of Dermatology
University of Campania
Caserta, Italy

Daniel Asz-Sigall
Department of Dermatology
Hospital General "Dr. Manuel Gea
 González"
Mexico City, Mexico

Kelati Awatef
Department of Dermatology
University Hospital Cheikh Khalifa, and
 the University Hospital Mohammed VI
Faculty of Medicine, Mohammed VI
 University of Health and Sciences
Casablanca, Morocco

Michelle S. Bach
University of Texas at Austin, Dell Medical
 School
Austin, Texas, USA
and
Department of Dermatology
Boston Medical Center
Boston, Massachusetts, USA

Anna Balato
Department of Dermatology
University of Campania
Caserta, Italy

Robert Baran
University of Franche-Comté, France, Nail
 Disease Center
Cannes, France

Asli Bilgic
Department of Dermatology and
 Venereology
Akdeniz University, Faculty of Medicine
Antalya, Türkiye

Luis Enrique Cano-Aguilar
Department of Dermatology
Hospital General "Dr. Manuel Gea
 González"
Mexico City, Mexico

Jade Conway
Department of Dermatology
Weill Cornell Medicine
New York, NY, USA

Eduardo Corona-Rodarte
Department of Dermatology
Instituto Dermatológico de Jalisco "Dr José
 Barba Rubio"
Zapopan, Mexico

Vishal Gaurav
Department of Dermatology and STD
All India Institute of Medical Sciences
New Delhi, India

Chander Grover
Department of Dermatology and STD
University College of Medical Sciences
New Delhi, India

Eckart Haneke
Department of Dermatology
Inselspital, University of Berne
Bern, Switzerland

Roderick Hay
King's College London
London, UK

Matilde Iorizzo
Private Practice
Bellinzona, Switzerland

Marta Kurzeja
Department of Dermatology
Medical University of Warsaw
Warsaw, Poland

Pauline Lecerf
Department of Dermatology, Brugmann
    and Saint Pierre University Hospitals
Université Libre de Bruxelles
Brussels, Belgium

André Lencastre
Central Lisbon Hospital Centre
Lisbon, Portugal

Shari Lipner
Department of Dermatology
Weill Cornell Medicine
New York, NY, USA

Agnieszka Michalczyk
Department of Dermatology
Medical University of Warsaw
Warsaw, Poland

Julia Nowowiejska
Department of Dermatology and
    Venereology
Medical University of Bialystok
Bialystok, Poland

Francesca Pampaloni
Department of Dermatology
University of Bologna
Bologna, Italy

Marcel C. Pasch
Department of Dermatology
Radboud University Medical Center
Nijmegen, The Netherlands

Vincenzo Piccolo
Department of Dermatology
University of Campania
Caserta, Italy

Bianca Maria Piraccini
Department of Dermatology
IRCCS Azienda Ospedaliero-Universitaria
    di Bologna
Bologna, Italy
and
Department of Medical and Surgical
    Sciences Alma Mater Studiorum
University of Bologna
Bologna, Italy

Luca Rapparini
Department of Dermatology
IRCCS Azienda Ospedaliero-Universitaria
    di Bologna
Bologna, Italy
and
Department of Medical and Surgical
    Sciences Alma Mater Studiorum
University of Bologna
Bologna, Italy

Bertrand Richert-Baran
Brugmann & Saint Pierre
University Hospitals
Universite Libre de Bruxelles, Belgium

Lidia Rudnicka
Department of Dermatology
Medical University of Warsaw
Warsaw, Poland

Ditte Marie L. Saunte
Department. of Allergy, Dermatology and
    Venereology
Herlev and Gentofte Hospital
Gentofte, Denmark

Michela Starace
Department of Dermatology
IRCCS Azienda Ospedaliero-Universitaria
    di Bologna
Bologna, Italy

Anna Waśkiel-Burnat
Department of Dermatology
Medical University of Warsaw
Warsaw, Poland

Elizabeth Yim
Division of Dermatology
University of Texas at Austin, Dell Medical
    School
Austin, Texas, USA

Part 1

Nails

1

Epidemiology

André Lencastre

1.1 Introduction

The most common nail disease, onychomycosis or tinea unguium, is a fungal nail infection that primarily affects the toenails and less often the fingernails [1–3]. Onychomycosis causes nail thickening and (discoloration dyschromia), often with separation of the nail plate from the bed (onycholysis), and may also affect the surrounding skin.

Due to its reported frequency and the relatively unspecific appearance of the nail changes caused by onychomycosis, it is the commonest differential diagnosis when a patient complains of nail disease. Furthermore, fungal superinfection can occur in a vulnerable dystrophic nail, as *locus minoris resistentiae*, when afflicted by another otherwise unrelated condition (e.g. inflammatory nail disease, trauma) [4,5].

Onychomycosis epidemiology is the study of its distribution, causes and specific regional variations within the world's population. Overall, it is the most common globally widespread nail disorder. Its prevalence varies among different populations. Prevalence estimates vary considerably in the general human population, with higher rates among older individuals, diabetics and those with compromised immune systems.

1.1.1 Risk Factors

Several factors increase the risk of developing onychomycosis. Furthermore, some of these same factors can also specifically reduce treatment success and increase the risk of recurrence after treatment, making onychomycosis a hard-to-treat, chronic condition, further contributing to a larger group of hosts. Risk factors for onychomycosis include:

Age: The incidence of onychomycosis increases with age, primarily due to inherently slower nail growth [6], difficulties in grooming nails and surrounding skin, long-standing and repeated nail trauma, reduced blood/lymphatic circulation, increased comorbidities (that can lead to further impair the immune system), immunosenescence [7] and cumulative exposure to fungi over time [5,8]. Even though children will uncommonly present with onychomycosis, likely due to the absence or lesser frequency of the aforementioned age-related risk factors, it definitely occurs [9–11]. Childhood onychomycosis is therefore a diagnosis to be considered and oftentimes an indicator of a coinfected parent or household member [12,13].

Gender: Men are more likely to be affected by toenail onychomycosis, and onychomycosis in general than women. This may be due to occupational or lifestyle factors

DOI: 10.1201/9781003381648-2

such as increased exposure to fungi in communal areas like locker rooms, gyms, pools and other facilities used for physical activities [5,8,14]. However, women more often will present with fingernail onychomycosis, since women have histori- cally been more involved in household activities [5]. Nevertheless, some studies have found no statistical difference in the prevalence of onychomycosis between groups [5]. Other studies allude to the opposite [15,16]. This may, in part, be attrib- utable to a higher tendency to seek medical care by women [17,18]. Geographically different cultural habits, between groups, in regard to footwear, bathing habits, occupation and participation in sports, may also be a factor [2].

Occupation and Lifestyle: Certain occupations and hobbies, like those involving pro- longed exposure to water or direct contact with fungi, can increase the risk of developing onychomycosis. Sports practitioners are at an increased risk of trau- matic nail disease and exposure to contaminated environments [8,19,20].

Personal Hygiene and Footwear: Poor foot hygiene, inadequate drying of feet, or shar- ing contaminated items like towels or nail clippers can contribute to the spread of fungal infections [21]. Damp, occlusive and closed footwear can also provide a lasting reservoir for infected skin material and fungal development [2].

Climate and Environment: Warm and humid conditions such as those found on tropi- cal climates provide a favourable environment for fungal growth. Rural environ- ments and cultural habit may favour the use of comfortable aerated open footwear. However, for those wearing shoes in a more urban setting and meeting occupa- tional expectations, high humidity, increased sweating and exposure to more humidity can contribute to the development of onychomycosis [15].

Comorbidities: Individuals with diabetes have a further risk of developing onychomy- cosis due to compromised blood circulation and a weakened immune system [5]. People with conditions such as HIV/AIDS and those undergoing immunosuppres- sive therapy or chemotherapy have a higher susceptibility to fungal infections, including onychomycosis [5]. Obesity has also been reported as an additional risk factor [22].

Trauma: Nail trauma, such as injuries, repetitive microtrauma or drug side effects, can (as previously stated) alter the nail structure or growth and facilitate fungal infection [5].

Other Nail Diseases: Patients with psoriasis may have a higher risk of onychomycosis [5].

Concomitant Neighbouring/Distant Skin Mycosis: Tinea pedis plantaris and tinea pedis interdigitalis are risk factors for nail infections and commonly co-occur with ony- chomycosis [8,23]. Onychomycosis can spread to the fingernails on the (usually dominant) hand that manipulates other infected body sites such as the feet or the toenails (in this instance acquiring the name two-feet-one-hand syndrome).

Genetic Predisposition: Beyond the interplay between all the above-mentioned envi- ronmental and host factors, an individual susceptibility to dermatophytosis must also be mentioned. Several candidate genes, responsible for skin homeostasis, in the innate immune response or fungi detection may be involved [24,25].

1.1.2 Fungal Agents

Onychomycosis is predominantly caused by dermatophytes, a group of fungi that commonly infect the skin, hair and nails. The most common dermatophyte species associated with onychomycosis (60%–70%) are *Trichophyton rubrum* and *Trichophyton mentagrophytes* [8]. Non-dermatophyte moulds such as *Scopulariopsis brevicaulis*, *Acremonium* spp., *Aspergillus* spp., *Fusarium* spp. and *Neoscytalidium* spp. can also cause nail infections, although less frequently. Yeast onychomycosis is mainly caused by *Candida* spp. in individuals whose fingernails are constantly immersed in water [1].

More attention has been given towards the prevalence of mixed infections by dermatophytes and non-dermatophyte moulds which have probably gone underestimated in the past [26].

Fungal pathogens responsible for onychomycosis are typically acquired from the environment. They can be found in warm and humid places like swimming pools, locker rooms, saunas and communal showers. Direct contact with infected individuals or sharing personal items like socks, shoes or nail care tools can also contribute to transmission.

1.2 Worldwide Epidemiology of Onychomycosis

It is difficult to determine the worldwide prevalence of onychomycosis. The average prevalence is currently estimated to be around 4.3% based on European and North American population studies only. Other world regions are lacking sufficient data [27].

Further research and surveillance efforts are therefore needed to obtain more comprehensive and up-to-date epidemiological data for each region. The prevalence and types of onychomycosis can vary geographically. While certain patterns and risk factors for onychomycosis are observed globally, there can be regional variations in prevalence and causative agents. The specific epidemiology of onychomycosis in each part of the world can be influenced by unique factors, including climate, culture, socioeconomic conditions and healthcare access.

1.3 Regional Variations in Onychomycosis Epidemiology

Studies on onychomycosis epidemiology in a specific region are of importance because of the constant change of both environmental and genetic factors, evolution of rural and urban communities, and transfer of pathogens due to migration [28]. Data reported in such studies might offer a better insight into onychomycosis risk factors and help tailor prevention and intervention programs.

However, as stated before, prevalence studies are scarce and probably most needed in certain geographical regions such as sub-Saharan Africa [29]. Furthermore, the distribution and prevalence are not static but change under the influence of various forces such as climate change, migration and developments in prophylaxis and therapy [2].

To specifically address regional epidemiological variations in onychomycosis, efforts should focus on increasing awareness among healthcare providers and the general population, improving access to healthcare services and conducting more research. Geographical and populational onychomycosis variations may depend less on geographical and/or continental borders, but more on the interplay between risk factors dependent on lifestyle and cultural habits, and relative distribution between rural and urban areas and different climate zones. Future studies should clearly address and identify these issues.

1.3.1 North America

In 1979, a large-scale population-based U.S. study reported a prevalence of 2.18%, using clinical examination as the criterion [30]. In spite of slight variation across U.S. and Canadian regions, global prevalence rates are estimated to be higher, ranging from 8.7% to 13.8% and likely to be increasing [8,14,31]. The risk factors associated with onychomycosis are similar to those observed globally, including age, gender (higher prevalence in males), diabetes, immunodeficiency, and occupational or lifestyle factors.

In Gupta et al.'s large Canadian multicentre extension study, dermatophytes (71.9%), particularly *T. rubrum* followed by *T. mentagrophytes*, were the predominant causative agents when compared with non-dermatophyte moulds (20.9%) and yeast (7.6%) [14].

Due to paucity of evidence, it is hard to estimate or comment on the relative impact between different cultural or socioeconomic factors within the North American populations and the prevalence of onychomycosis, if any. Regional differences in lifestyle, residence in rural or urban areas and among diverse climates have not been substantially characterized.

1.3.2 Europe

Due to differences in study design, the prevalence range is broader when compared with the US and is reported from as low as 0.5% to as high as 20% [5,11,22,23,32–34]. Although regional differences in climate have to be considered, the same general risk factors apply as cultural tendencies regarding footwear, occupational habits and hobbies may be shared. Again, dermatophytes are the main causes, mostly *T. rubrum*, followed by *T. mentagrophytes* [17]. Yeasts and non-dermatophyte moulds appear to be the second and third most common causative fungal subgroups.

1.3.3 South America

Onychomycosis is also prevalent in South America, although very limited data are available for this region as a whole. A recent systematic review of mostly clinical over population studies, by Pereira et al., places estimated prevalence rates of dermatophyte onychomycosis around 25% [35]. Climate and environmental factors, such as warm and humid conditions prevalent in some areas, may contribute to the high prevalence. Dermatophytes, especially *T. rubrum*, *T. mentagrophytes* and *T. interdigitale*, are the primary causative agents [18,35]. A recent study has highlighted the higher rate of mixed infections detected in Brazil [26].

1.3.4 Asia, Australia and Oceania

Onychomycosis is recognized as a common condition in many Australasian countries. The prevalence rates can vary across different populations and this vast region, ranging from 0.5% to 25% [36–39]. Again, risk factors for onychomycosis may significantly vary between climates and different environmental factors (warm and humid conditions), choices in footwear, socioeconomic factors (poor living conditions and limited access to clean water), comorbidities and rural vs. urban living. Cultural practices, such as walking barefoot or wearing sandals, provide higher ventilation and therefore reduce fungal development on the feet [40], probably overcoming an expected increased exposure and likelihood of infection from contaminated surfaces [41].

The predominant causative agents are dermatophytes, although there may be regional variations [36–38].

1.3.5 Africa

Onychomycosis is considered a common condition in Africa, although specific data on prevalence are limited. Prevalence rates can range from 2% to 15% in different African populations [42].

Onychomycosis is rarely reported in studies coming from rural, tropical African regions. Noticeably, however, data are relatively scarce compared to other regions of the world, placing doubt whether this is due to lower prevalence, underdiagnosis or publication bias regarding neglect for this condition. Beyond diverse climate conditions and environmental factors, risk factors for onychomycosis in Africa include socioeconomic factors (such as poor living conditions, limited access to clean water, inadequate sanitation and hygiene), comorbidities (such as HIV/AIDS) and lower access to healthcare [43,44].

Dermatophytes, especially *Trichophyton* spp., are the primary causative agents in certain African regions [45]; however, a higher rate of yeast fingernail onychomycosis in female patients is the main nail condition reported in others [16,46].

1.4 Conclusion

Accurately measuring the prevalence of onychomycosis is crucial to estimate the burden of this disease and predict the potential demand for medical treatment and its economic impact.

Several challenges affect our understanding of the epidemiology of onychomycosis:

1. *Limited Data*: Despite onychomycosis being a common condition, there is a lack of comprehensive epidemiological data from diverse regions, reported in a consistent fashion. More studies and surveillance efforts are needed to better understand this disease, its risk factors, preference for certain population groups and regional variations.

2. *Study Design*: A homogeneous methodology should ideally be followed and reported on [47]. More population-based studies are needed over clinical (hospital-based) studies [14,27]. Beyond well-known established risk factors, better knowledge of different patient study groups can be obtained regarding their occupation, habitual footwear, social setting and perhaps their location in regard to Köppen–Geiger climate classification system [48].

3. *Underdiagnosis and Lack of Awareness*: Onychomycosis is already often underdiagnosed in Europe and North America. Limited awareness among both healthcare providers and the general population throughout the world can contribute to this issue. The condition may be neglected or mistaken for other nail disorders, delaying proper diagnosis and treatment, and this may relate to erroneous estimates of the disease.

4. *Healthcare Access*: Limited access to healthcare facilities and diagnostic tests, particularly in rural, remote or otherwise poorer areas, can hinder early diagnosis and appropriate management of onychomycosis. Without a grasp on the true epidemiology of onychomycosis, it is harder to issue advice on public health policy changes.

References

1. Gupta A, Stec N, Summerbell R, et al. Onychomycosis : a review. *J Eur Acad Dermatol Venereol.* 2020;34(9):1972–90.
2. Gill D, Marks R. A review of the epidemiology of tinea unguium in the community. *Australas J Dermatol.* 1999;40(1):6–13.
3. Vlahovic TC. Onychomycosis: evaluation, treatment options, managing recurrence, and patient outcomes. *Clin Pod Med Surg.* 2016;33(3):305–18.
4. Schiavo A, Lo, Ruocco E, Russo T, et al. Locus minoris resistentiae : an old but still valid way of thinking in medicine. *Clin Dermatol.* 2014;32(5):553–6.
5. Maraki S, Mavromanolaki VE. Epidemiology of onychomycosis in Crete, Greece: a 12-year study. *Mycoses.* 2016;59(12):798–802.
6. Bean WB. Nail growth: 30 years of observation. *Arch Intern Med.* 1974;134(3):497–502.
7. Sinikumpu SP, Jokelainen J, Haarala AK, et al. The high prevalence of skin diseases in adults aged 70 and older. *J Am Geriatr Soc.* 2020;68(11):2565–71.
8. Ghannoum MA, Hajjeh RA, Scher R, et al. A large-scale North American study of fungal isolates from nails: the frequency of onychomycosis, fungal distribution, and antifungal susceptibility patterns. *J Am Acad Dermatol.* 2000;43(4):641–8.
9. Vestergaard-Jensen S, Mansouri A, Jensen LH, et al. Systematic review of the prevalence of onychomycosis in children. *Pediatr Dermatol.* 2022;39(6):855–65.
10. Song G, Zhang M, Liu W, Liang G. Children onychomycosis, a neglected dermatophytosis: a retrospective study of epidemiology and treatment. *Mycoses.* 2023;66(5):448–54.
11. Kromer C, Celis D, Hipler UC, et al. Dermatophyte infections in children compared to adults in Germany: a retrospective multicenter study in Germany. *JDDG – J Ger Soc Dermatology.* 2021;19(7):993–1001.
12. Philpot CM, Shuttleworth D. Dermatophyte onychomycosis in children. *Clin Exp Dermatol.* 1989;14(3):203–5.
13. Chang P, Logemann H. Onychomycosis in children. *Int J Dermatol.* 1994;33(8):550–1.
14. Gupta AK, Gupta G, Jain HC, et al. The prevalence of unsuspected onychomycosis and its causative organisms in a multicentre Canadian sample of 30 000 patients visiting physicians' offices. *J Eur Acad Dermatol Venereol.* 2016;30(9):1567–72.
15. Lupa S, Seneczko F, Jeske J, et al. Epidemiology of dermatomycoses of humans in central Poland. Part IV. Onychomycosis due to dermatophytes. *Mycoses.* 1999;42(11–12):657–9.
16. Sylla K, Tine RCK, Sow D, et al. Epidemiological and mycological aspects of onychomycosis in Dakar (Senegal). *J Fungi.* 2019;5(2):2–11.
17. Powell J, Porter E, Field S, et al. Epidemiology of dermatomycoses and onychomycoses in Ireland (2001-2020): a single-institution review. *Mycoses.* 2022;65(7):770–9.
18. Relloso S, Arechavala A, Guelfand L, et al. Onicomicosis: estudio multicéntrico clínico, epidemiológico y micológico. *Rev Iberoam Micol.* 2012;29(3):157–63.
19. Haneke E. Epidemiology and pathology of onychomycoses. In: Nolting S, Korting HC, editors. *Onychomycoses.* Berlin: Springer; 1989. pp. 1–11.
20. Buder V, Augustin M, Schäfer I, et al. Prevalence of dermatomycoses in professional football players: a study based on data of German Bundesliga fitness check-ups (2013–2015) compared to data of the general population. *Hautarzt.* 2018;69(5):401–7.
21. Jazdarehee A, Malekafzali L, Lee J, et al. Transmission of onychomycosis and dermatophytosis between household members: a scoping review. *J Fungi.* 2022;8(1):60.
22. Burzykowski T, Molenberghs G, Abeck D, et al. High prevalence of foot diseases in Europe: results of the Achilles project. *Mycoses.* 2003;46(11–12):496–505.
23. Perea S, Ramos MJ, Garau M, et al. Prevalence and risk factors of tinea unguium and tinea pedis in the general population in Spain. *J Clin Microbiol.* 2000;38(9):3226–30.
24. Gnat S, Łagowski D, Nowakiewicz A. Genetic predisposition and its heredity in the context of increased prevalence of dermatophytoses. *Mycopathologia.* 2021;186(2):163–76.

25. Vinh DC. Of mycelium and men: inherent human susceptibility to fungal diseases. *Pathogens*. 2023;12(3):456.
26. Gupta AK, Taborda VBA, Taborda PRO, et al. High prevalence of mixed infections in global onychomycosis. *PLOS ONE*. 2020;15:1–8.
27. Sigurgeirsson B, Baran R. The prevalence of onychomycosis in the global population – a literature study. *J Eur Acad Dermatology Venereol*. 2014;28(11):1480–91.
28. Bontems O, Fratti M, Salamin K, et al. Epidemiology of dermatophytoses in Switzerland according to a survey of dermatophytes isolated in Lausanne between 2001 and 2018. *J Fungi*. 2020;6(2):1–8.
29. Urban K, Chu S, Scheufele C, et al. The global, regional, and national burden of fungal skin diseases in 195 countries and territories: a cross-sectional analysis from the global burden of disease study 2017. *JAAD Int*. 2021;2:22–7.
30. Johnson ML, Johnson KG, Engel A. Prevalence, morbidity, and cost of dermatologic diseases. *J Am Acad Dermatol*. 1984;11(5 pt 2):930–6.
31. Elewski BE, Charif M. Prevalence of onychomycosis in patients attending a dermatology clinic in Northeastern Ohio for other conditions. *Arch Dermatol*. 1997;133(9):1172–3.
32. Sergeev A, Ivanoy O, Sergeev Y, et al. Epidemiology of onychomycosis in modern Russia: incidence is growing. *Mycoses*. 2002;45(S2):56.
33. Papini M, Piraccini BM, Difonzo E, et al. Epidemiology of onychomycosis in Italy: prevalence data and risk factor identification. *Mycoses*. 2015;58(11):659–64.
34. Svejgaard EL, Nilsson J. Onychomycosis in Denmark: prevalence of fungal nail infection in general practice. *Mycoses*. 2004;47(3–4):131–5.
35. De Oliveira Pereira F, Gomes SM, Da Silva SL, et al. The prevalence of dermatophytoses in Brazil: a systematic review. *J Med Microbiol*. 2021;70(3).
36. Shimoyama H, Satoh K, Makimura K, et al. Epidemiological survey of onychomycosis pathogens in Japan by real-time PCR. *Med Mycol*. 2019;57(6):675–80.
37. Kayarkatte MN, Singal A, Pandhi D, et al. Clinico-mycological study of onychomycosis in a tertiary care hospital – a cross-sectional study. *Mycoses*. 2020;63(1):113–18.
38. Song G, Zhang M, Liu W, et al. Epidemiology of onychomycosis in Chinese Mainland: a 30-year retrospective study. *Mycopathologia*. 2022;187(4):323–31.
39. Coloe S, Baird R. Dermatophyte infections in Melbourne: trends from 1961/64 to 2008/09. *Australas J Dermatol*. 2010;51(4):258–62.
40. Ramesh V, Reddy B, Singh R. Onychomycosis. *Int J Dermatol*. 1983;22(3):148–52.
41. Bhutani L, Mohapatra L, Kandhar K. Tinea pedis – a penalty of civilization. A sample survey of rural and urban population. *Mykosen*. 1971;7(6):335–6.
42. Djeridane A, Djeridane Y, Ammar-Khodja A. Epidemiological and aetiological study on tinea pedis and onychomycosis in Algeria. *Mycoses*. 2006;49(3):190–6.
43. Ezomike NE, Ikefuna AN, Onyekonwu CL, et al. Epidemiology and pattern of superficial fungal infections among primary school children in Enugu, south-east Nigeria. *Malawi Med J*. 2021;33(1):21–7.
44. Coulibaly O, L'Ollivier C, Piarroux R, et al. Epidemiology of human dermatophytoses in Africa. *Med Mycol*. 2018;56(2):145–61.
45. Araya S, Abuye M, Negesso AE. Epidemiological characterization of dermatomycosis in Ethiopia. *Clin Cosmet Investig Dermatol*. 2021;14:83–9.
46. Zafindraibe N, Tsatoromila F, Rakotoarivelo Z, et al. Onychomycosis: experience of the laboratory of parasitology-mycology of CHU-Joseph Ravoahangy Andrianavalona, Antananarivo, Madagascar. *Pan African Med Journal*. 2021;40:176.
47. Chabasse D. Peut-on chiffrer la fréquence des onychomycoses? *Ann Dermatol Venereol*. 2003;130(12):1222–30.
48. Beck HE, Zimmermann NE, McVicar TR, et al. Present and future Köppen-Geiger climate classification maps at 1-km resolution. *Sci Data*. 2018;5:1–12.

2

Anatomy of the Nail

Asli Bilgic

2.1 Introduction

The nail unit refers to the entire complex structure including nail plate, surrounding tissues and components of vasculature, innervation and bone. It is not only an important aesthetic organ but also an essential element of diagnosis for some systemic diseases or for the protection of fingertips along with improving fine touch and digit movements.

The nail unit development begins at the 10th embryonal week on the fingertips and at the 17th embryonal week on the tips of the toes. It appears as a result of a series of complex mesenchymal-ectodermal interactions, involving the signalling of Wnt and bone morphogenetic proteins (BMPs). These pathways regulate the crosstalk between the epidermis and mesenchyme, and control and manage the induction and differentiation of nails. The nails reach the tips of the fingers at the 32nd gestational week and the tips of the toes at the 36th embryonal week [1–5].

The nail unit consists of four key structures (nail plate, nail matrix, nail bed and perionychium [proximal, lateral and distal nail folds]) along with several other specific components (such as lunula, cuticle, distal free edge of the plate, onychodermal band and hyponychium) which will be discussed in this chapter (Figure 2.1).

2.2 Nail Plate

The nail plate is the hard, semi-transparent, visible part of the nail. It protects the sensitive nail matrix and bed and supports the function of the fingers and toes with its special physical characteristics such as being hard and difficult to break but also being elastic and bendable. Its structure is also resistant to chemicals.

The nail plate is mainly produced by the nail matrix. It has three horizontal layers: a dorsal lamina, the intermediate lamina and a ventral layer from the nail bed. The thin dorsal layer of the nail plate (0.08–0.1 mm thick) consists of flattened onychocytes and has a smooth surface. The hardness and sharpness of the nail plate is attributed to this portion which is produced by the proximal matrix. The intermediate layer is composed of less flattened onychocytes, is much thicker (0.3–0.5 mm thick) and is produced by the distal matrix. Nail flexibility and elasticity are attributed to this second layer. The ventral layer (0.06–0.08 mm thick), on the other hand, that is sometimes not regarded as a true layer is mainly nail bed keratin and it provides the necessary adhesion of the nail plate to the nail bed [4–10].

DOI: 10.1201/9781003381648-3

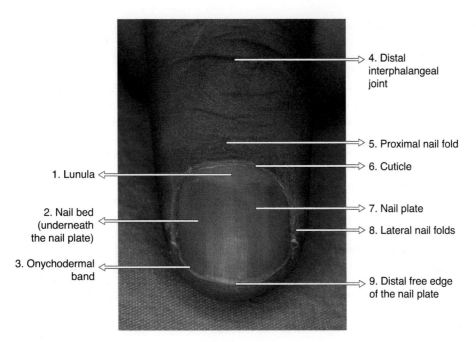

1. Lunula
2. Nail bed (underneath the nail plate)
3. Onychodermal band
4. Distal interphalangeal joint
5. Proximal nail fold
6. Cuticle
7. Nail plate
8. Lateral nail folds
9. Distal free edge of the nail plate

FIGURE 2.1
The key structures of the nail unit.

The nail plate over the nail bed is normally transparent and colourless. However, because of the reflection of the pinkish colour of the nail bed, the nail plate seems to have a light pink colour. On the other hand, the distal free edge of the nail plate has often more yellowish white colour due to the increased refraction because of the solid–gas interface in this area.

The thickness of the nail plate is determined by the length of the matrix and it increases from the proximal to the distal end. The nails are approximately 0.5–0.75 mm thick. The thickness differs between fingernails and toenails as well as between genders. The thumb nail is the thickest on the hands and the thickness of the nail decreases in other fingers. The average nail plate thickness is 0.5 mm in women and 0.6 mm in men. With aging, the size of the onychocytes in the plate increases and growth rate decreases which result in thicker nail plates [11–14].

The nail plate is limited by the proximal and the lateral nail folds. There is a continuous forward movement of the nail plate starting from the proximal nail matrix until the distal free edge; all along the way, the nail plate is strongly adherent to the nail bed. Fingernails grow approximately 0.1 mm/day or 3 mm/month. Toenails grow slower than the fingernails. Complete regrowth of a fingernail may require 6 months, and a toenail requires 12–18 months [10].

The nail plate is slightly curved in both longitudinal and transverse directions (but more markedly curved in the transverse direction which is mostly affected by the shape of the distal phalanx). The curvature of the nails is also affected by genetic factors, gender, age, mechanical forces and neurogenic factors. Transverse convexity is more prominent in toenails than in fingernails and it leads to better attachment of the plate to the nail bed [15–17]. The longitudinal curvature on the other hand is believed to be the result of faster proliferation rate of the proximal matrix cells compared to the distal matrix. The outer surface of the nail plate is smooth and shiny, but often might have a number of longitudinal ridges. The ventral surface also has longitudinal ridges and indentations due to the complementary ridges on the upper aspect of the nail bed which adds firmness to the attachment of the plate and nail bed [18].

Nails are composed of 80%–85% sulphur-rich hard keratins and densely packed flattened onychocytes along with 10%–20% basic soft keratins. There are cross-linked disulphide bonds which give the nail its physical and chemical stability. There is also a significant proportion of amino acids (cysteine, glutamic acid, arginine, aspartic acid, serine and leucine) found in the nail plate. In terms of minerals and electrolytes, various amounts were found including elements like calcium but also sodium, potassium, magnesium, iron, copper, zinc, phosphorus, selenium, sulphur and several others. However, the hardness of the nail is not related to the amount of calcium but rather to the tight bonding of the nail plate layers. Nail plate also contains 0.1%–1% of lipids, where cholesterol is the primary lipid component, and 7%–12% of water which changes according to environmental factors. The softness of the nail increases with the amount of hydration [19–22].

The shape of the nail depends on different factors. As previously mentioned, the length of the nail matrix usually defines the thickness of the nail plate, and the breadth of the matrix determines the width of the nail plate (narrow or broad nails). Moreover, the length of the nail bed defines the nail plate length (long or short nails), and the shape of the underlying bone contributes to the shape of the nail [22–24].

2.3 Nail Matrix

The nail matrix, located at the base of the nail, is the main source of the nail plate (Figure 2.2). Like the epidermis, it has a dividing basal layer where keratinocytes are produced, and the evaluation of these keratinocytes involves differentiation, hardening and becoming dead keratinized cells that form the nail plate. There is an eosinophilic area known as the keratogenous zone, where proliferating keratinocytes from the nail matrix start to express hard keratins. However, the maturation of these keratinocytes is different from the epidermis as there is no granular layer (keratohyalin formation) in the nail matrix [14,22].

In the mid-part of the nail matrix, the matrix epithelium is thicker with long, oblique rete ridges, distally oriented. Near the nail bed, the distal matrix epithelium is thinner. Laterally, the matrix rete ridges are less marked. In the distal matrix, the connective tissue is loose and oedematous; on the other hand, in the proximal matrix and the nail bed, it has dense collagen bundles, vertically oriented and firmly connecting the nail apparatus to the periosteum. Because the nail matrix is located beneath the proximal nail fold and cuticle, it is closely related to the extensor tendon insertion near the distal interphalangeal joint. The distance between the apex of the matrix and the extensor tendon insertion is around 1–1.4 mm [25–28]. Recent anatomic studies even show that the proximal limit of the matrix of the great toe and fingers somehow overlaps with the terminal extensor tendons until its distal bony insertion [29–31]. On the other hand, the lateral corners of the matrix and the proximal portion of the nail plate extend more proximally on both lateral sides and these often are called horns of the matrix [10,32] (Figure 2.3).

The normal nail matrix especially proximal matrix has around 200 melanocytes per mm^2 in the suprabasal layer, whereas they decrease moving towards the distal nail matrix.

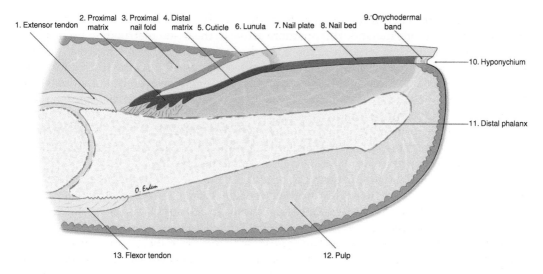

FIGURE 2.2
Lateral schematic view of the nail unit showing the important structures and components of the nail unit: 1, extensor tendon; 2, proximal matrix; 3, proximal nail fold; 4, distal matrix; 5, cuticle; 6, lunula; 7, nail plate; 8, nail bed; 9, onychodermal band; 10, hyponychium; 11, distal phalanx; 12, pulp; 13, flexor tendon.

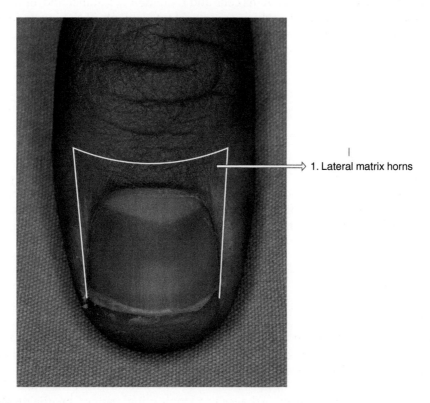

FIGURE 2.3
The extent of lateral nail horns. These lateral corners of the matrix extend more proximally on both lateral sides: 1, lateral matrix horns.

However, they are much more numerous in the matrix than in the nail bed (absent to $50/mm^2$). Furthermore, melanocytes are more active in the distal matrix than in the proximal matrix, and they are larger and more dendritic as well [25,33–37]. Especially in fair skinned individuals and Caucasians, melanocytes are mostly dormant and functionally inactive; thus, melanonychia is not a common finding. However, in individuals with Fitzpatrick skin type 3–6, these melanocytes although being in normal distribution might produce enough melanin to cause physiological nail pigmentation [18,38].

The matrix is the primary area where nail growth originates; thus, injuries or damage to the matrix often might result in changes or deformities in the growing nail. The health of the nail matrix is essential for maintaining the overall nail health.

There are specifically two skin stem cell populations in the nail unit where regeneration occurs. The main ones are the highly proliferative stem cells of the nail matrix. They have a fast cycle and mostly renew the nail plate. The other stem cell population is the slow-cycling stem cells of the proximal nail fold. These can both play a role in regenerating the peri-nail epidermis under normal conditions and contribute to the nail if there is an injury [5].

There is also the concept of immune privilege (IP) which is also seen in the nail matrix similar to important tissues such as hair follicle bulge, the eyes and the central nervous system. It protects these tissues from the exaggerated inflammation or autoimmune reaction. In the nail matrix, it was shown that there is a downregulation of MHC class I expression on both keratinocytes and melanocytes, remarkably downregulated expression of MHC class II and CD209 by Langerhans cells and reduction in number and/or function of natural killer cells and mast cells which are important elements of the innate immunity; meanwhile increased local expression of transforming growth factor-β1 and α-melanocyte stimulating hormone was demonstrated which are potent immunosuppressants [2].

2.4 Lunula

The lunula is the visible pale half-moon-shaped area at the base of the nail, near the proximal nail fold. It's actually a part of the nail matrix that's visible through the nail plate. The lunula is more pronounced in some individuals and less visible in others. It is most commonly visible on the thumbs, middle fingers and great toes. The shape of the lunula often outlines the shape of the distal margin of the nail plate [22,39].

2.5 Nail Bed

The nail bed is the tissue lying underneath 75%–85% of the nail plate between the distal edge of the lunula and the onychodermal band (hyponychium) (Figure 2.4). The blood vessels in the nail bed give the nail its pinkish colour. There are longitudinally running capillaries which are arranged one above the other in 4–6 rows under the nail bed epithelium. Splinter haemorrhages, haemorrhages in a longitudinal pattern, are the result of this specific arrangement appearing after the nail bed capillary is damaged [18].

Nail bed is composed of epithelium that is flat-topped and longitudinally ridged, and has regular parallel alignment of ridges. The nail bed epithelium cells keratinize very

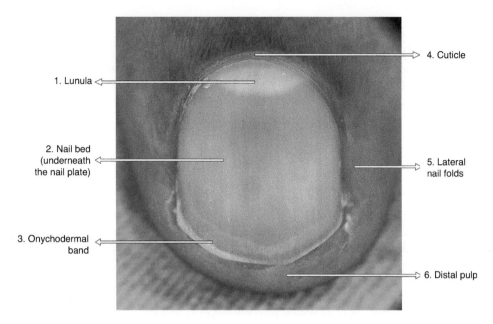

FIGURE 2.4
Upper dermoscopic view of the nail unit. Cuticle and lunula is more apparent along with the pinkish nail bed. Just before the distal free edge of the nail plate, the different hue shows the onychodermal band area: 1, lunula; 2, nail bed (underneath the nail plate); 3, onychodermal band; 4, cuticle; 5, lateral nail folds; 6, distal pulp.

gradually throughout the extension of the nail bed and disappear at the onychodermal band, where the epithelium is thicker and there is a high collection of onycholemmal keratin. The nail bed epithelium is not regarded as a self-generating and independent structure, and it derives from the matrix epithelium. The transition between the nail matrix and the nail bed is barely visible on histologic examination [9,25]. Nail bed epithelium has stratified cells that are no more than two or three cells thick, do not show mitoses and transform from living keratinocyte to dead ventral nail plate cells. This ventral layer of the plate originating from the nail bed moves distally with the nail plate growth. Nail bed keratin expression lacks the terminal differentiation of the normal skin. It is suggested that this could be due to the nail plate acting as a cornified epithelium, thus the nail bed does not produce its own [9,17].

2.6 The Nail Mesenchyme

Onychodermis is the term sometimes used for the specialized nail mesenchyme which lies below the nail matrix and nail bed over the distal phalanx. However, the nail unit has no actual epidermis and dermis similar to the skin; thus, this term is not accepted by experts. The nail mesenchyme is the connective tissue without apparent subcutaneous fat, lying over the distal phalangeal bone. It has a complex innervation network along with a strong vascular network including multiple glomus bodies that are arteriovenous anastomoses. Furthermore, it hosts Merkel cells and Meissner bodies with many nerve endings. These specific components play an important role on the sensitivity, fine touch and fine movements of the digit pulp [22,25].

2.7 Nail Folds

The nail unit is surrounded on three sides by the proximal and lateral nail folds. This whole area is called the paronychium. The epithelium of these nail folds is similar to normal skin, differing only by the absence of pilosebaceous units [18].

2.8 Proximal Nail Fold (Posterior Nail Fold)

The proximal nail fold covers the base of the nail plate and it's an extension of the skin surrounding the nail. It is formed by a dorsal and a ventral part: the dorsal portion continues distally with the skin of the digit. It has a similar epidermis to the digit skin except for the absence of hair and sebaceous glands (no pilosebaceous follicles). The undersurface or ventral surface of the proximal nail fold is on the other hand covered by a thin and flattened epidermis with a well-developed stratum granulosum [18,25]. The proximal nail fold also contains keratin-producing cells which provide support as a protective barrier. The proximal nail fold is not meant to be pushed back or trimmed like the visible cuticle, as this can lead to irritation, inflammation and potential damage to the nail matrix.

2.9 Cuticle (Eponychium)

The terms "proximal nail fold" and "cuticle" are sometimes used interchangeably, although the cuticle normally describes the thin layer of dead skin cells seen at the base of the nail. On the other hand, the proximal nail fold is the living tissue covering the area. The cuticle is actually an extension of the horny layer of both the dorsal as well as the ventral skin of the proximal nail fold. It appears slightly translucent and might have a whitish-yellowish colour differentiating it from the surrounding skin. It may be more prominent in some individuals and less visible in others. It protects the nail matrix and provides a barrier preventing debris, dirt and pathogens from entering the area and thus a barrier to potential infections. It also helps to seal the nail plate and to prevent excessive water loss from the nail matrix [18].

2.10 Lateral Nail Folds

These are folds of skin on the sides of the nail plate bordering the nail plate on each side extending from the base of the nail to the tip and contribute to the strong attachment of the nail plate to the nail bed. They are typically more prominent in the toes than in the fingers. The primary function of the lateral nail fold is to protect the area beneath the nail plate.

2.11 The Free Edge of the Nail Plate

The distal free edge of the nail plate is the part of the nail plate which can be trimmed. This part has often an opaque structure due to the increased refraction at the solid–gas interface at the free edge of the nail plate.

2.12 Onychodermal Band and Hyponychium

The onychodermal band is the keratinized distal part of the nail bed that functions as an attachment for the distal nail plate where the nail plate separates from the fingertip. It has a different colour compared to the rest of the nail bed and is usually seen as a transverse band of 1–1.5 mm in darker pink colour in Caucasians. However, its colour could change due to skin type, compression or with diseases [17,22]. It functions as a barrier and plays an important role in maintaining the health and protection of the underlying nail bed.

The terms "hyponychium" and "onychodermal band" are often used interchangeably. However, hyponychium defines the area of skin located distal to the onychodermal band between the distal free edge of the nail and the fingertip. It's the point where the nail plate separates from the underlying nail bed and is the transition between the nail bed epithelium and the skin of the digital pulp. Like any other epidermal areas, hyponychium undergoes normal keratinization and exhibits a granular layer and eccrine glands [18].

2.13 Vascular Supply

2.13.1 Arterial

The radial and ulnar arteries supply deep and superficial palmar arcades that act as a large anastomosis between these two vessels. The main blood supply to the nail unit comes from the proper digital arteries which are a branch of these arteries. The proper digital arteries branch proximal to the distal interphalangeal joint, supply blood to the nail unit from both the paired volar (palmar) as well as dorsal proper digital arteries, but the volar arteries are the main suppliers. These arteries create three arcades: distal subungual arcade, proximal subungual artery (arcade), and superficial arcade (Figure 2.5). The dorsal nail fold arch (superficial arcade) could be found just distal to the distal interphalangeal joint. It supplies the nail fold and extensor tendon insertion. The subungual region is supplied by the distal and proximal subungual arcades, arising in turn from an anastomosis of the palmar arch and the dorsal nail fold arch. The palmar arch is located beneath the maximal padding of the finger pulp in a protected area [9,10,40–42].

Nail fold vessels and capillary network are similar to normal skin; however, the capillary loops of the proximal nail fold follow a parallel pattern to the skin surface and are usually visible throughout their length. In normal conditions they are in uniform size and their number is around 30 per 5 mm. They can be seen with a video dermatoscope at 20× or more magnifications or with a capillaroscopy machine. The changes in number and

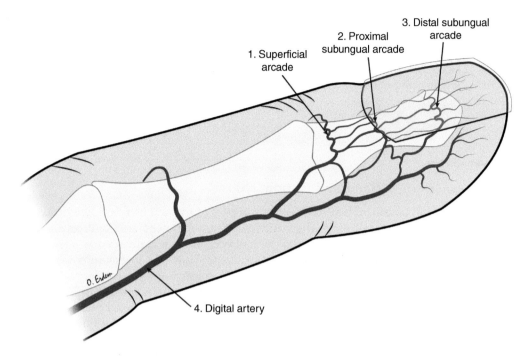

FIGURE 2.5
The arterial supply of the nail unit: 1, superficial arcade; 2, proximal subungual arcade; 3, distal subungual arcade; 4, digital artery.

shape of these capillaries and loops might point out to connective tissue diseases. On the other hand, the capillaries of the nail matrix and the hyponychium have similarity with skin capillaries [17].

2.14 Venous

The venous system of the nail unit has more variability although being less abundant. Venous drainage of the fingers is by deep and superficial systems. The deep venous drainage of the nail unit mostly follows parallel paths to the arterial supply. Superficially, there exist the dorsal and palmar digital veins, consisting of many arcades on the dorsal and palmar surface of the digit with connecting oblique and transverse anastomosis. Dorsal veins are larger with a more prominent branching network, and palmar veins are often smaller [10,17].

The superficial dorsal veins are the main channels for venous drainage from the fingertip. The venules first appear at the sides of the fingernail and unite together proximal to the nail bed, forming a central vein. This dorsal central vein runs in the dorsal midline of the distal phalanx. This vein divides into two or three branches and then unite again after passing over the distal interphalangeal joint [10,41,43–47]. A recent study from Japan showed that in the fingers, the distance from the nail lunula edge to the central vein at the eponychial level was about 5 mm and that from the central vein to the adjacent vein at the DIP joints was about 6–8 mm [48].

The vascular structure of the nail unit is complex with many arteriovenous anastomoses in the distal digit, from simple shunts to the complex glomus bodies. Glomus bodies are small neurovascular bodies creating arteriovenous anastomosis bypassing the intermediary capillary bed. Because of their rich nerve supply, they function as regulators of capillary circulation, especially in temperature changes of weather or surroundings [10,17].

2.15 Lymphatic Drainage

Compared to the arterial and venous supply of the nail unit, the lymphatic drainage of the nail unit is rather unknown and less studied.

2.16 Nerve Supply

Nerve innervation is important for maintaining sensitivity, touch perception, pain detection, and controlling the underlying muscles and blood vessels.

The nail unit receives one branch from the dorsal digital nerve and one ventral branch from the palmar digital nerve. The periungual soft tissues are innervated by the dorsal branches running at the sides of the flexor tendon and with the dorsal neurovascular bundle. They follow a path over the distal interphalangeal joint to the proximal nail fold, and the dorsal digital nerves are probably the main innervation for most of the digits although there are some debates about the type of innervation of digit tips. Generally, the thumb, little finger as well as the toe tips have their innervation from the dorsal nerves; meanwhile the index, middle and ring fingertips are innervated by the palmar digital nerves [17,18]. The palmar digital nerve follows the proper digital artery across the distal interphalangeal joint, lying palmar and medial to the artery. Distal to the distal interphalangeal joint, the digital nerve gives three major fascicles supplying the nail unit, the digit tip and the pulp of the distal digit. Nerve endings were shown to lie close to the epithelial surface, especially in the nail folds [18,22].

2.17 Distal Phalanx

The entire nail unit is fixed to the underlying terminal phalanx. The skeletal component of the nail unit consists of the terminal phalangeal bone and the distal interphalangeal joint (DIF). The phalanx has a head, a widened proximal base and a tapered shaft. The shape and size of the bone effect the shape and size of the nail [23,49]. The DIF joint is a hinged synovial joint and laterally stabilized by lateral ligaments and also by lateral branches of both the extensor and flexor tendons.

2.18 Conclusion

To conclude, it is obvious that the nail unit is a complicated organ and has important roles and functions. It is essential to know the nail unit anatomy and to use the terminology correctly for not only evaluating the nail diseases and performing nail surgeries but also recording in the patients' files, monitoring and sharing these in scientific publications.

Acknowledgements

I would like to thank Assist. Prof. Ozan Erdem, MD, Consultant Dermatologist, Department of Dermatology and Venereology, Istanbul Medeniyet University for the illustrations and arrangement of photos used in this chapter.

References

1. Moore KL, Persaud TV. *Integumentary System*. In: Keith L Moore, TVN Persaud, Mark G Torchia (eds.) *The Developing Human: Clinical Oriented Embryology*. 10th ed. Saunders Elsevier Philadelphia, USA; 2008:437–54.
2. Saito M, Ohyama M, Amagai M. Exploring the biology of the nail: an intriguing but less-investigated skin appendage. *J Dermatol Sci*. 2015;79(3):187–93.
3. Blaydon DC, Ishii Y, O'Toole EA et al. The gene encoding R-spondin 4 (RSPO4), a secreted protein implicated in Wnt-signaling, is mutated in inherited anonychia. *Nat Genet*. 2006;38:1245–7.
4. McCarthy DJ. Anatomic considerations of the human nail. Review. *Clin Podiatr Med Surg*. 2004;21(4):477–91.
5. Pulawska-Czub A, Pieczonka TD, Mazurek P, et al. The potential of nail mini-organ stem cells in skin, nail and digit tips regeneration. *Int J Mol Sci*. 2021;22(6):2864.
6. Johnson M, Comaish JS, Shuster S. Nail is produced by the normal nail bed: a controversy resolved. *Br J Dermatol*. 1991;125(1):27–9.
7. Johnson M, Shuster S. Continuous formation of nail along the bed. *Br J Dermatol*. 1993;128(3):277–80.
8. González-Serva A. Normal nail anatomy, normal nail histology, and common reaction patterns. In: Rubin AI, Jellinek NJ. Daniel III CR, et al., editors. *Scher and Daniel's Nails, Diagnosis, Surgery, Therapy*, 4th ed. Springer, Switzerland; 2018:39–83.
9. Dawber RPR, Science of the nail apparatus. In: Baran R, Dawber RPR, Haneke E, et al., editors. *A Text Atlas of Nail Disorders Techniques in Investigation and Diagnosis*, 3th ed. Taylor & Francis, London, UK; 2003:1–10.
10. Haneke E. Surgical anatomy of the nail apparatus. *Dermatol Clin*. 2006;24:291–6.
11. Johnson M, Shuster S. Determinants of nail thickness and length. *Br J Dermatol*. 1994;130(2):195–8.
12. Hamilton J, Terada H, Mestler G. Studies of growth throughout the lifespan in Japanese: growth and size of nails and their relationship to age, sex, heredity, and other factors. *J Gerontol*. 1955;10:401–16.
13. Zaias, N. *The Nail in Health and Disease*. Springer Science & Business Media; 2012.

14. de Berker D, Mawhinney B, Sviland L. Quantification of regional matrix nail production. *Br J Dermatol.* 1996;134:1083–9.
15. Jung JW, Kim KS, Shin JH, et al. Fingernail configuration. *Arch Plast Surg.* 2015;42(6):753–60.
16. Sano H, Ogawa R. Clinical evidence for the relationship between nail configuration and mechanical forces. *Plast Reconstr Surg Glob Open.* 2014;2(3):115.
17. de Berker D. Nail anatomy. *Clin Dermatol.* 2013;31(5):509–15.
18. Haneke E. Development, structure and function of the nail. In: Haneke E, editor. *Histopathology of the Nail, Onychopathology.* CRC Press, Taylor & Francis Group, Boca Raton; 2017:1–19.
19. Lynch M, O'Guin W, Hardy C, et al. Acidic and basic hair/nail ("hard") keratins: their colocalization in upper cortical and cuticle cells of the human hair follicle and their relationship to "soft" keratins. *J Cell Bio.* 1986;103:2593–606.
20. Gupchup GV, Zatz J. Structural characteristics and permeability properties of the human nail: a review. *J Cosmet Sci.* 1999;50:363–85.
21. Baswan S, Kasting GB, Li SK, et al. Understanding the formidable nail barrier: a review of the nail microstructure, composition and diseases. *Mycoses.* 2017;60(5):284–95.
22. de Berker DAR, Baran R, Science of the nail apparatus. In: Baran R, de Berker DAR, Holzberg M, et al., editors. *Baran & Dawber's Diseases of the Nails and Their Management,* 4th ed. John Wiley & Sons, Ltd, UK; 2012:1–51.
23. Parrinello JF, Japour CJ, Dykyj D. Incurvated nail. Does the phalanx determine nail plate shape? *J Am Podiatr Med Assoc.* 1995;85(11):696–8.
24. Fleckman P, McCaffrey L. Structure and function of the nail unit, In: Rubin AI, Jellinek NJ. Daniel III CR, et al., editors. *Scher and Daniel's Nails, Diagnosis, Surgery, Therapy,* 4th ed. Springer, Switzerland; 2018;8:39–83.
25. André J, Sass U, Richert B, et al. Nail pathology. *Clin Dermatol.* 2013;31(5):526–39.
26. Shum C, Bruno RJ, Ristic S, et al. Examination of the anatomic relationship of the proximal germinal nail matrix to the extensor tendon insertion. *J Hand Surg.* 2000;25:1114–17.
27. Schweitzer TP, Rayan GM. The terminal tendon of the digital extensor mechanism: part I, anatomic study. *J Hand Surg.* 2004;29:898–902.
28. Reardon CM, McArthur PA, Survana SK, et al. The surface anatomy of the germinal matrix of the nail bed in the finger. *J. Hand Surg. Br.* 1999;24:531–3.
29. Palomo López P, Becerro de Bengoa Vallejo R, López López D, et al. Anatomic relationship of the proximal nail matrix to the extensor hallucis longus tendon insertion. *J Eur Acad Dermatol Venereol.* 2015;29(10):1967–71.
30. Palomo-López P, Becerro-de-Bengoa-Vallejo R, López-López D, et al. Anatomic association of the proximal fingernail matrix to the extensor pollicis longus tendon: a morphological and histological study. *J Clin Med.* 2018;7(12):465.
31. Palomo-López P, Losa-Iglesias ME, Becerro-de-Bengoa-Vallejo R, et al. Anatomic and histological features of the extensor digitorum longus tendon insertion in the proximal nail matrix of the second toe. *Diagnostics.* 2020;10(3):147.
32. Jellinek NJ, Rubin AI. Lateral longitudinal excision of the nail unit. *Dermatologic Surg.* 2011;37:1781–5.
33. de Berker D, Dawber RPR, Thody A, et al. Melanocytes are absent from normal nail bed; the basis of a clinical dictum. *Br J Dermatol.* 1996;134:564.
34. Perrin C, Michiels JF, Pisani A, et al. Anatomic distribution of melanocytes in normal nail unit: an immunohistochemical investigation. *Am J Dermatopathol.* 1997;19:462–7.
35. Higashi N. Melanocytes of nail matrix and nail pigmentation. *Arch Dermatol.* 1968;97:570–4.
36. Higashi N, Saito T. Horizontal distribution of the DOPA-positive melanocytes in the nail matrix. *J Invest Dermatol.* 1969;53:163–5.
37. Tosti A, Cameli N, Piraccini BM, et al. Characterization of nail melanocytes with anti-PEP1, anti-PEP8, TMH-1, and HMB-45 antibodies. *J Am Acad Dermatol.* 1994;31:193–6.
38. Hashimoto K. Ultrastructure of the human toenail. I. Proximal nail matrix. *J Invest Dermatol.* 1971;56:235–46.

39. Cohen PR. The lunula. *J Am Acad Dermatol.* 1996;34(6):943–53.
40. Soon PS, Arnold MA, Tracey DJ. Paraterminal ligaments of the distal phalanx. *Acta Anat.* 1991;142(4):339–46.
41. Chaudakshetrin P, Kumar VP, Satku K, et al. The arteriovenous pattern of the distal digital segment. *J Hand Surg Br.* 1988;13(2):164–6.
42. Smith DO, Oura C, Kimura C, et al. Artery anatomy and tortuosity in the distal finger. *J Hand Surg Am.* 1991;16(2):297–302.
43. Lucas GL. The pattern of venous drainage of the digits. *J Hand Surg Am.* 1984;9(3):448–50.
44. Moss SH, Schwartz KS, von Drasek-Ascher G, et al. Digital venous anatomy. *J Hand Surg Am.* 1985;10(4):473–82.
45. Nyström A, von Drasek-Ascher G, Fridén J, et al. The palmar digital venous anatomy. *Scand J Plast Reconstr Surg Hand Surg.* 1990;24(2):113–19.
46. Lhuaire M, Wavreille G, Hivelin M, et al. Venous system mapping of the digits and the hand: an anatomical study and potential surgical applications. *JPRAS Open.* 2022;33:171–83.
47. Berritto D, Iacobellis F, Rossi C, et al. Ultra high-frequency ultrasound: new capabilities for nail anatomy exploration. *J Dermatol.* 2017;44(1):43–46.
48. Tsumura T, Matsumoto T, Matsushita M, et al. Examination of the dorsal finger vein anatomy using a vein visualization device. *J Hand Surg Asian Pac.* 2020;25(3):291–5.
49. Baran R, Juhlin L. Bone dependent nail formation. *Br J Dermatol.* 1986;114:371–5.

3

Clinical Patterns of Onychomycosis Correlated with Routes of Entry*

Robert Baran and Roderick Hay

3.1 A Revised Classification of Onychomycosis

In 1990, Zaias devised a classification of onychomycosis based on the clinical appearances of onychomycosis [1]. This was later revised in 2002 [2] and in this section further revisions are made to this enlarged clinical classification taking into account the current state of knowledge and new clinical descriptions and findings (Figure 3.1). The purpose of this classification is to provide a framework to assist selection of treatment, the likely prognosis and to evaluate new diagnostic methods. It is important to recognize, though, that sometimes more than one of these patterns can coexist in the same nail.

There are several guiding principles to this approach.

- The observed clinical patterns and their evolution in fungal nail disease provide a clue to the type of infection present. But these cannot be relied on to make a definitive diagnosis of fungal infection using clinical grounds alone, although when taken together with other observed findings, such as the unilateral involvement of the nails on one hand and palm together with both soles, they can provide powerful clues to the diagnosis. The clinical features should be linked with the results of laboratory investigation.

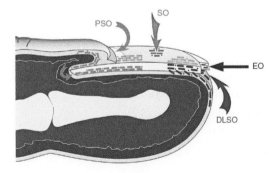

FIGURE 3.1
Routes of fungal nail infection.

---

* This chapter includes figures from Rigopoulos R, Baran R, Onychomycosis, in Baran R, Rigopoulos D, Grover C, Haneke E, eds, *Nail Therapies: Current Clinical Practice* 2E, CRC Press, 2021.

DOI: 10.1201/9781003381648-4

- Visualizing fungal elements by direct microscopy also does not identify the type of fungus involved, except that with appropriately trained observers, yeasts can usually be differentiated from dermatophytes and occasionally a *Microascus* (*Scopulariopsis*) infection can be identified by the nature of the spores produced in nail or dematiaceous fungal causes may be suspected by their dark colouration.
- A reliable identification of the causal agent can only be made by culture or molecular diagnostic tools.
    - It is sometimes difficult to isolate fungi in culture even from nails which are positive in direct microscopy.
    - The culture or molecular identification of a particular fungus is not always a proof of its aetiological role. Therefore, to determine whether a fungus is a commensal or if it is truly responsible for nail dystrophy, additional criteria and clinical correlation are necessary.
    - Finally, histopathology usually and reliably demonstrates whether a fungus is invasive or merely colonizing subungual debris.
- Species identification cannot be made from direct microscopy, and since different causative organisms may require different therapy, a culture or molecular diagnostic test should always be performed. Since about one third of mycological studies may be negative, a nail biopsy may be appropriate.
- Though certain patterns of nail involvement are characteristic of individual species, generally the clinical appearances caused by one species of fungus is indistinguishable from that caused by another.
- The invading fungus produces proteolytic enzymes which enable it slowly to digest the nail keratin. Initially, the nail becomes detached from the nail bed, thus changing its colour to a creamy-white and opaque shade. Thereafter, reactive hyperkeratosis develops on the underside of the nail plate leading to thickening.
- Fungal infection is by far the commonest nail disorder which will respond to specific treatment and therefore it is important not to miss the diagnosis.

3.2 Classification of Onychomycosis

1. *Distal and lateral subungual onychomycosis (DLSO)*
    This is the most common clinical presentation of onychomycosis. There are different clinically recognizable components.

    1.1 Subungual hyperkeratosis (Figure 3.2)

    1.2 Onycholysis (Figure 3.3)

    1.3 Paronychia (Figure 3.4)

    1.4 Melanonychia (Figure 3.5)

2. *Proximal subungual onychomycosis (PSO)*
    This is a rare type of onychomycosis that may occur equally often in the toenails, as in the fingernails. It is mostly caused by *Trichophyton. rubrum* and is common in untreated HIV/AIDS.

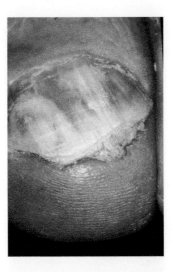

FIGURE 3.2
DLSO Subungual hyperkeratosis.

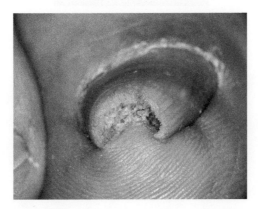

FIGURE 3.3
DLSO with Onycholysis.

2.1 With paronychia

    2.1.1 Presumed *Candida* paronychia (Figure 3.6). Here the organism is present either as a commensal or following on from colonization of a pre-existing paronychium caused by other pathologies such as irritant dermatitis.

    2.1.2 True *Candida* paronychia are rare and usually observed in chronic muco-cutaneous candidiasis (CMCC) or HIV positive subjects.

    2.1.3 Non-dermatophyte moulds may also cause paronychia and are also sometimes associated with leukonychia (e.g. *Fusarium, Neoscytalidium*) (Figure 3.7).

    2.1.4 Dermatophyte infection (rare)

2.2 Without paronychia

This type is called proximal subungual onychomycosis (PSO) or proximal white subungual onychomycosis (PWSO). There are three variants seen in dermatophyte infections and one associated with *Candida*.

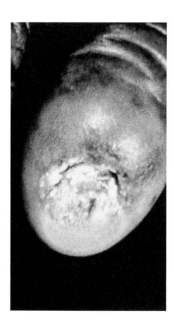

FIGURE 3.4
DLSO with Paronychium.

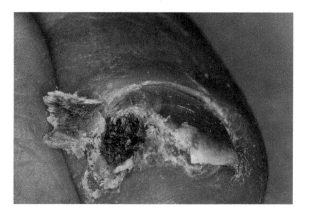

FIGURE 3.5
DLSO with melanonychia.

2.2.1 Classical PWSO that consists of white subungual patches appearing from beneath the proximal nail fold (Figure 3.8).

2.2.2 Proximal white transverse subungual onychomycosis (PTSO) presents as a PSO with atypical patterns: striate leukonychia are present as isolated or multiple bands (Figure 3.9). These are transverse subungual white strips, separated by zones of nail that are both clinically and histologically normal, affecting the same digit. Proximal to distal longitudinal leukonychia presenting with bands or streaks affecting a single digit is rare.

2.2.3 Acute PWSO. A rapidly developing form of PWSO is recorded in patients with HIV who usually have a CD4+ cell count of less than 450 cells/mm^3.

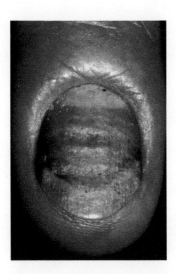

FIGURE 3.6
PSO (lateral) with Paronychium.

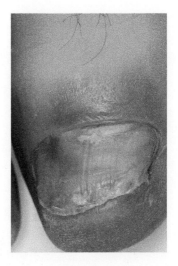

FIGURE 3.7
PSO with infection due to Fusarium.

This acute type of nail invasion involves several digits simultaneously (Figure 3.10).

2.2.4 *Candida* PWSO has been reported in chronic mucocutaneous candidiasis (CMCC)

2.2.5 A combination pattern is seen in AIDS patients where PWSO and SO may develop at the same time and spread rapidly to involve the nail plate.

3. *Superficial onychomycosis (SO)*

This type occurs primarily in the toenails and is usually caused by fungi of the *Trichophyton mentagrophytes* complex (90% of cases). Often the affected nail shows discrete patches of nail plate involvement, less commonly (see below) these are linear and transverse bands. The commonest pattern presents with white bands or

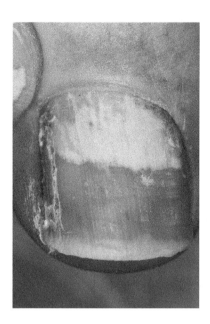

FIGURE 3.8
Classical PWSO.

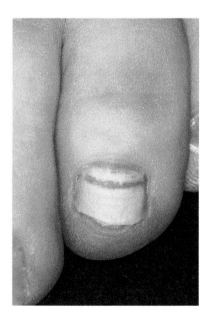

FIGURE 3.9
Proximal white transverse subungual onychomycosis (PTSO).

patches on the nail, superficial white onychomycosis (SWO). Sometimes the adjacent toe may overlap the affected nail plate.

3.1 Classical SWO type restricted to the visible nail plate (Figure 3.11). There is also a black variant.

3.2 Superficial white onychomycosis (SWO) originating under the proximal nail fold (Figure 3.12)

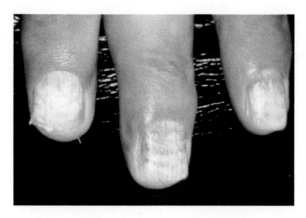

FIGURE 3.10
Acute Proximal White Subungual Onychomycosis (PWSO).

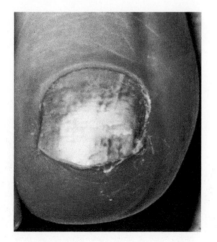

FIGURE 3.11
Classical Superficial White Onychomycosis SWO.

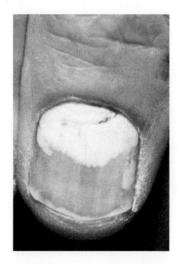

FIGURE 3.12
SWO from Proximal Nail Fold.

3.3 Acute (rapidly developing) SWO (Figure 3.13)

3.4 Superficial transverse pattern (STO) – this shows superficial transverse bands (Figure 3.14)

3.5 SWO with deep invasion (Figure 3.15). The nail plate usually appears thickened but the deep invasion is confirmed by histopathology.

3.6 Three Mixed patterns with three variants:

    3.6.1 SWO with DLSO

    3.6.2 SWO with PSO

    3.6.3 SWO associated with histologically restricted involvement of the ventral aspect of the nail plate (bipolar type)

4. *Endonyx onychomycosis (EO). (due to* Trichophyton soudanense *and* violaceum*)*

These fungi may also cause other forms of onychomycosis (Figure 3.16). The infection penetrates the nail keratin instead of infecting the nail bed. It is not

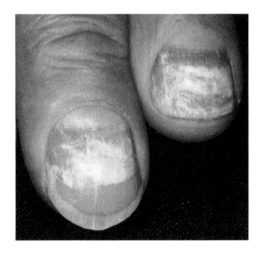

FIGURE 3.13
Acute SWO.

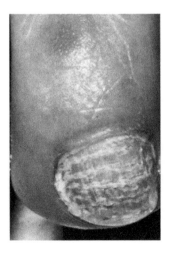

FIGURE 3.14
Superficial transverse pattern (STO).

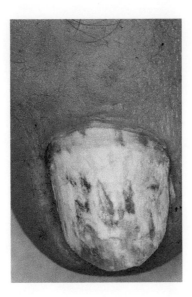

FIGURE 3.15
SO with deep invasion.

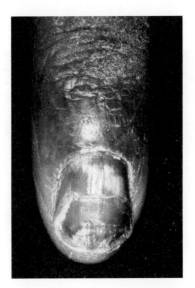

FIGURE 3.16
Endonyx onychomycosis (EO).

common but usually caused by *T. soudanense* and *T. violaceum*, both of which have high affinity for keratin.

5. *Total dystrophic onychomycosis (TDO)*

    5.1 TDO presents secondary to other forms (Figure 3.17). This is the end result of the complete progression of any of the above-mentioned clinical patterns of onychomycosis. It leads to dystrophy of the whole nail plate.

    5.2 Primary TDO (CMCC) (Figure 3.18). This only occurs in patients with chronic mucocutaneous candidiasis, a primary immunodeficiency syndrome. It develops rapidly and the original location of the nail infection is not apparent.

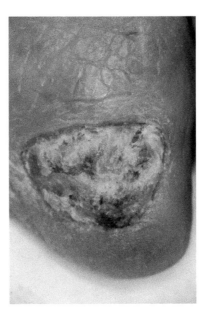

FIGURE 3.17
Total Dystrophic Onychomycosis (TDO).

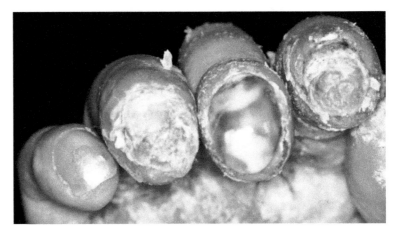

FIGURE 3.18
Primary Total Dystrophic Onychomycosis (TDO).

3.3 Distal and Lateral Onychomycosis

This is the commonest pattern of nail infection and is particularly associated with derma-tophytes such as *T. rubrum*. As the infection proceeds unchecked, the demarking front of the infection extends progressively towards the proximal nail and fold areas. The expand-ing lesion is usually irregular and there may be more rapid progression of the infection along the lateral borders of the nail. It is accompanied by onycholysis and thickening of the nail plate with the appearance of eroded and crumbly areas of the nail plate which become softer. The colour is usually pale to white, although in some areas there may be a brownish tinge. Fungal melanonychia is seen with some dermatophytes such as melanizing strains of *T. rubrum* as well as some *Neoscytalidium* infections.

3.3.1 Proximal Subungual Onychomycosis

Proximal subungual onychomycosis, which is rare in healthy adults, was recorded as a significant problem among HIV positive individuals before the availability of combination antiretroviral therapy but it is also sometimes seen in organ transplant recipients. Given the acute presentation observed in the former and characterized by multi-nail involvement, often symmetrically distributed on the nails, the potential existence of an indirect route for spread, e.g. lymphatic and blood-borne, has been suggested [3]. The connection between *Fusarium* nail infection and digital cellulitis followed by disseminated *Fusarium* infections in severely neutropenic patients is suggestive of a route from the nail into the general circulation, under rare circumstances.

Superficial (white) onychomycoses are most commonly caused by the dermatophyte, *T. mentagrophytes* var. *interdigitale*, whose keratinolytic enzymes can metabolize the hard keratins on the nail surface. However, this classical understanding is challenged by the less straightforward realities, such as the deep invasion in certain so-called superficial forms, dorsal and ventral bipolar manifestations of the nail, the appearance of a proximal superficial variety originating under the periungual fold, and a variety consisting of multiple transverse trabeculae that relate some superficial onychomycoses to proximal subungual onychomycoses through a common fungal penetration process.

3.3.1.1 Clinical Presentation

Proximal subungual onychomycosis has specific clinical characteristics. Clinical changes appear under the periungual fold and extend towards the distal region. This can occur in both fingers and toes.

The stratum corneum of the ventral surface of the periungual fold is traditionally considered the site of primary fungal invasion in this variety. The fungus thence progresses to the nail matrix and the ventral part of the nail.

From a clinical perspective, the first sign is usually a white spot appearing under the nail plate, smooth and transparent, with a normal cuticle adhering to it. The leukonychia gradually extends towards the distal nail region. The ventral region of the periungual fold may reveal a defined fungal, dermo-epidermal, focus, a histological feature described by Zaias [1].

Usually affecting the toes, superficial fungal leukonychia presents as small white islands with distinct boundaries that progressively cover the entire nail surface, making it both irregular and softer than normal. These lesions easily crumble on scratching the site with a blunt curette or scissor blade. When observed late, the lesions sometimes take on a yellowish colour.

In addition to this clinical presentation, proximal subungual onychomycosis can present in other patterns:

- Proximal localized leukonychia, usually on one nail
- Simple or multiple transverse leukonychial bands. In this case, the bands are separated by normal appearing nail (clinically and/or histologically).

- Acute form of proximal subungual leukonychia observed in HIV+ patients with CD4 counts below 450 cells/mm^3. This variety is characterized by simultaneous invasion of multiple nails, usually at the same level.

It has been suggested that there is a potential role for deep lymphatic involvement in certain types of onychomycoses [3]. To support this argument, there is evidence of deep dissemination of dermatophytes in the rare syndrome originally described from North Africa where there is deep dermatophytosis in individuals with inherited *CARD9* gene mutations [4,5]. These individuals may develop deep organ and lymph node dermatophyte infection. A further case report showed a biopsy confirmed deep dermatophyte infection apparently originating from a toenail lesion in a patient presenting with unilateral lymphatic obstruction, accompanied by secondary spread of the dermatophyte infection from the foot and toes with a dermal granuloma below the homologous knee [6].

Both examples suggest that sequestration of dermatophytes from the normal epidermal site to lymphatics can occur, under unusual but very specific circumstances [6–8]; to what extent this or similar mechanism can explain the severe and rapid-onset PSO in HIV/AIDS patients remains to be seen.

3.3.2 Superficial Onychomycoses

Superficial onychomycoses constitute a less common form of nail involvement than the distal and lateral subungual form. However, there are important practical therapeutic implications in this form of nail invasion.

There are subvarieties of superficial fungal leukonychia:

- The classic form, confined to the visible part of the nail surface
- A variant of the preceding type but originating from the proximal nail and appearing from beneath the cuticle and often invading multiple toes simultaneously
- Superficial onychomycosis with secondary deep penetration into the nail keratin. Piraccini and Tosti described this as a form seen in childhood as well as in the immunosuppressed [9].
- A rare striate variety, consisting of superficial whitish transverse bands, single or multiple, separated by normal coloured nail. These bands originate from under the nail fold.

3.3.3 Mixed Forms of Onychomycosis

Finally, there are true mixed forms where superficial onychomycosis and other forms of onychomycosis coexist – three variants have been recorded:

- White patches on the dorsal nail plate associate with distal and lateral subungual onychomycosis [9].
- Superficial bands of leukonychia emerging from under the proximal nail fold and combined with PWSO presenting as transverse or arcuate lines or patches with an arcuate distal border or as a non-homogeneous opaque nail plate. This has been described in HIV positive and immunocompetent patients [10–13].
- A combined type where the white patches on the dorsum of the nail plate are accompanied by histological involvement of the ventral aspect of the nail plate – but without clinical signs of deep invasion.

The apparent origin of infection from beneath the posterior nail fold in some variants of SWO and the possible overlap with PWSO may be grounds for arguing that they share a common route of infection in some cases. This has therapeutic implications as except for the classical type of SWO where only the visible portion of the nail plate is involved, the other variants need to be treated with systemic antifungals alone or in combination with topical antifungal nail lacquers. The source of infection in those types that originate from beneath the proximal nail fold presumably reflects a similar origin of infection as proximal subungual onychomycosis itself.

- Mixed forms, which can be divided into two groups:
  1. Bipolar form, where white patchy spots on the nail surface accompany proximal subungual fungal invasion, affecting the ventral surface of the nail plate.
  2. The association of superficial discrete white patches appearing below the cuticle and proximal subungual onychomycosis presents as opaque white nail or transverse white lines or white patches with the distal limit following the lunular crescent shape.

3.3.3.1 Practical Daily Implications

The aforementioned discussion shows that superficial fungal leukonychia, once thought to be distinctive due to its superficial invasion mode compared to the distal and lateral or proximal subungual mycotic invasion, exhibits forms that may appear together with the proximal subungual variety. This suggests a possible common origin in certain cases.

This has significant implications for the treatment of onychomycoses. Apart from the classic form of superficial onychomycosis where only the visible part of the nail is affected and topical treatment is indicated, all other varieties require systemic treatment in addition to topical antifungals.

The prospect of other possible fungal penetration route in proximal and superficial subungual onychomycoses is particularly interesting, as this condition affects not only HIV+ patients but also organ transplant recipients and immunocompetent individuals. Some of these types including those associated with HIV usually require longer courses of oral treatment and failure rate is high.

Superficial white onychomycosis itself is generally caused by either dermatophytes such as *T. mentagrophytes* var. *interdigitale* or non-dermatophytes such as *Acremonium*, *Fusarium* or *Aspergillus* species. In their review of white superficial onychomycosis, Piraccini and Tosti [9] described the clinical features of 79 cases and pointed out the relationship between age and immunosuppression and different patterns of infection.

3.4 Other Clinical Patterns Seen in Onychomycosis

a. Subungual dermatophytoma

For some time it has been recognized that opaque streaks and localized areas of onychomycosis were associated with treatment failure [14]. It has been suggested that this should be called "subungual dermatophytoma" [15]. Clinically, either a dense white linear streak or a round white, yellow/brown or opaque area is seen (Figure 3.19). The nail overlying these areas shows onycholysis and when it is cut

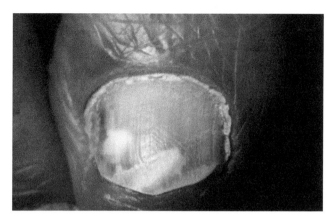

FIGURE 3.19
Subungual dermatophytoma presenting as a lateral streak.

back, a thick spongy hyperkeratotic mass is revealed. Histology of this mass may contain a densely packed clump of irregular dermatophyte hyphae or these may be more sparsely distributed. This mass is soft and can be scraped away. This may represent a form of fungal biofilm, although some only contain sparse fungal hyphae. Clinically, a dermatophytoma may present as a longitudinal yellow band ("spike") or as a round yellow or white area in the nail plate. Dermatophytomas are most commonly seen in DLSO forms of onychomycosis.

b. Melanonychia

Melanin produced by fungi can sometimes infiltrate the nail plate [16]. This has been recorded with both DLSO and SO forms of infection. The causes are varied, with melanizing strains of *T. rubrum* (Figure 3.20) and *Neoscytalidium* species both

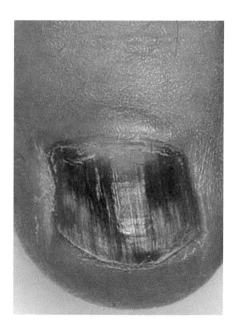

FIGURE 3.20
Melanonychia (*T.rubrum*).

reported as causing this phenomenon. This may involve substantial areas of the nail or patches on the surface, but rarely the melanonychia may present with pigmented linear streak in the nail plate [17].

c. Two feet–one hand syndrome

It has long been recognized that onychomycosis of the hand due to dermatophytes may present unilaterally [18]. Often this is accompanied by scaling on the palm of that hand where there is onychomycosis yet both feet are affected by onychomycosis and dry type dermatophytosis of the soles. The unilateral hand distribution is therefore a clue to the cause. The reasons for this are unclear but it does not seem to be associated with handedness [19].

3.5 Unusual Forms of Onychomycosis due to *Candida* Involving Fingernails

Although most patterns of *Candida* infection of the nail fit with the classification scheme outlined above, *Candida* infection starting at or shortly after birth may have some unusual features. Congenital cutaneous candidiasis (CCC) is a rare intra-uterine fungal infection of the dermis and epidermis acquired by vertical transmission and vaginal colonization by *Candida* species [20,21]. Most cases are seen at birth, but onset can be as late as 6 days, usually presenting as a diffuse maculopapular eruption on the skin that later evolves to pustules with subsequent desquamation. The rash is often generalized, affects palms and soles (differentiating it from miliaria and erythema toxicum neonatorum), and spares mucous membranes and diaper area. CCC may also present with signs of systemic infections, such as respiratory distress, especially in infants who are preterm. There may also be fingernail involvement, by invasion of nail plate via the hyponychial epithelium, that manifests as onychomadesis – complete nail shedding of the proximal sector, with yellowish hyperkeratotic bands and paronychia. Nail dystrophy may be present at birth or develop as late as after 6 weeks of life. This condition must be distinguished from other non-infectious causes of congenital nail dystrophy, such as congenital pachyonychia or onychodysplasia [21].

References

1. Zaias N. *The Nail in Health and Disease*, 2nd ed. Norwalk, CT: Appleton & Lange; 1990.
2. Baran R, Hay RJ, Tosti A, Haneke E A new classification of onychomycosis. *Br J Dermatol.* 1998;139:567–71.
3. Hay RJ, Baran R. Deep dermatophytosis: rare infections or common, but unrecognised complications of lymphatic spread? *Curr Opin Infect Dis.* 2004;17:77–9.
4. Hadida E, Schousboe A, Sayag J. Dermatophyties atypiques. *Bull Soc Fr Dermatol Syphiligr.* 1966;73:917–25.
5. Lanternier F, Pathan S, Vincent QB, et al. Deep dermatophytosis and inherited CARD9 deficiency. *N Engl J Med.* 2013;369:1704–14.
6. Mayou S, Calderon RA, Hay RJ, Goodfellow A. Deep dermatophyte infection. *Clin Exp Dermatol.* 1987;12:385–8.

7. Baran R, McLoone N, Hay RJ. Could proximal white subungual onychomycosis be a complication of systemic spread? The lessons to be learned from Maladie dermatophytique and other deep infections. *Br J Dermatol.* 2005;153:1023–25.
8. Tjasvi T, Sharna VK, Sethuraman G. et al. Invasive dermatophytosis with lymph node involvement in an immunocompetent patient. *Clin Exp Dermatol.* 2005;30:506–8.
9. Piraccini BM, Tosti A. White superficial onychomycosis. *Arch Dermatol.* 2004;140:696–701.
10. Basuk PJ, Scher RK. Onychomycosis in graft versus host disease. *Cutis* 1987;40:237–41.
11. Baran R, Hay R, Perrin C. Superficial white onychomycosis revisited. *JEADV* 2004;18:569–71.
12. Gupta AK, Summerbell RC. Combined distal and lateral subungual and white superficial onychomycosis in the toenails. *JAAD* 1999;41: 938–44.
13. Keisman K, Knudsen EA, Pedersen C. White nails in AIDS/AKC due to *Trichophyton rubrum* infection. *Clin Exp Dermatol.* 1988;13:24–25
14. Hay RJ. Chronic dermatophyte infections. In: Verbov J., editors. *Superficial Fungal Infections.* Lancaster, UK: MTP Press Ltd; 1986. pp. 23–4.
15. Roberts DT, Evans EG. Subungual dermatophytoma complicating dermatophyte onychomycosis. *Br J Dermatol.* 1998;138:189–90.
16. Finch J, Arenas R, Baran R. Fungal melanonychia. *JAAD* 2012;66:830–41.
17. Badillet G. Mélanonychies superficielles. *Bull Soc Fr Mycol Med.* 1988;XVII(2):335–40.
18. Daniel CR 3rd, Gupta AK, Daniel MP, Daniel CM. Two feet-one hand syndrome: a retrospective multicenter survey. *Int J Dermatol.* 1997;36:658–60.
19. Hay RJ. Chronic dermatophyte infections. I. Clinical and mycological features. *Br J Dermatol.* 1982;106:1–7.
20. Colantonio S, Hedin E, Li HO, et al. Management of congenital cutaneous candidiasis in a healthy term baby: a case report. *SAGE Open Med Case Rep.* 2019;7:2050313X19876707. doi: 10.1177/2050313X19876707.
21. Tuoni C, Mazzatenta C, Filippi L. Congenital cutaneous candidiasis with nail involvement. *J Pediatr.* 2023;260:113470.

4

Clinical Differential Diagnosis of Fungal Nail Infections

Matilde Iorizzo and Marcel C. Pasch

Onychomycosis is so frequently encountered in daily practice that any nail dystrophy, especially one occurring in isolation, may be wrongly diagnosed. In addition, some entirely different dermatoses may cause similar nail alterations. This is due to the fact that the nail apparatus has a limited repertoire of reaction patterns and the nail plate covers and hides the very structures involved in the pathological process. Some examples are given below.

4.1 Distal Lateral Subungual Onychomycosis with Prominent Subungual Hyperkeratosis

This can be mimicked by several inflammatory nail conditions, characterized by their protracted and recalcitrant courses.

1. **Psoriasis** (Figure 4.1) is the skin disease that most often produces nail changes and can mimic onychomycosis.
   Subungual hyperkeratosis can be isolated or associated with onycholysis, leukonychia and distal splinter haemorrhages. As distortion and dystrophy of the nail plate may be seen in both onychomycosis and psoriasis, it may be impossible to diagnose psoriasis restricted to the nails on clinical grounds alone unless there is extensive pitting and/or the oil drop sign.

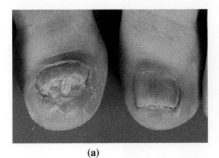
(a)

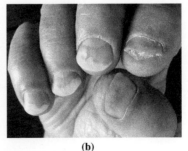
(b)

FIGURE 4.1
(a) Psoriasis of the toenails; (b) Psoriasis of the fingernails.

DOI: 10.1201/9781003381648-5

Psoriatic nails are said to be more susceptible to fungal infection. Hence dual infection is not exceptional in toenails [1,2].

2. Skin changes and nail features in **Reiter's syndrome** may be indistinguishable from those of patients with psoriasis. However, a brownish-red hue of the nail bed lesions may suggest this condition.

3. **Repeated microtrauma.** Epithelial hyperplasia of the subungual tissues may result from repeated trauma (Figure 4.2).

4. **Pityriasis rubra pilaris** (Figure 4.3). In adult acute-onset type I pityriasis rubra pilaris nail involvement usually presents as distal subungual hyperkeratosis with moderate thickening of the nail bed, splinter haemorrhages and longitudinal ridging.

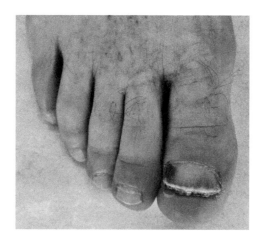

FIGURE 4.2
Repeated microtrauma.

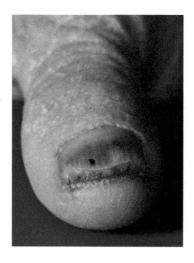

FIGURE 4.3
Pityriasis rubra pilaris.

5. **Norwegian (crusted) scabies** (Figure 4.4). The hyperkeratotic lesions are accompanied by large, psoriasis-like accumulations of scales under the nails and may resemble onychomycosis due to *Trichophyton rubrum*. The mites survive in these dystrophic nails and later colonize the skin, first around the nail plates; from there, they extend proximally. This type of scabies is most often seen in the old and infirm, the mentally ill and AIDS patients and during immunosuppression.

6. **Darier's disease** (Figure 4.5). In typical cases the nails have longitudinal subungual pink or white streaks or both, and distal wedge-shaped subungual keratoses.

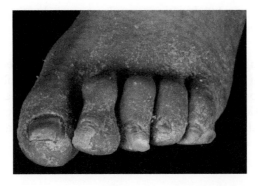

FIGURE 4.4
Scabies.

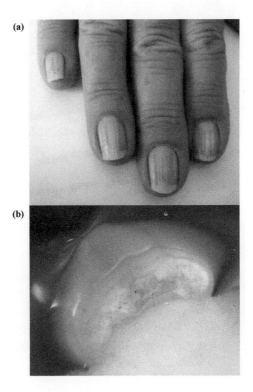

FIGURE 4.5
(a and b) Darier's disease.

7. **Lichen planus** (Figure 4.6). Usually there is a progressive thinning and fluting of the nail and marked subungual hyperkeratosis may lift the nail plate. It may therefore be associated with onycholysis which can sometimes be seen in isolation.

8. **Chronic contact dermatitis** (Figure 4.7). The cause of nail changes is obvious when the eczema has a periungual distribution. It may be difficult to recognize in atopic dermatitis, discoid eczema, etc. The modifications of the nail result from disturbances of the matrix. These may present as thickening, pitting and transverse ridging sometimes leading to shedding of the nail. Exudative skin disease may occur with any chronic condition involving this area.

9. **Erythroderma** (Figure 4.8). In chronic erythroderma due to Sézary syndrome, for example, nail changes are similar to those found in patients with type I pityriasis rubra pilaris.

10. **Pachyonychia congenita** (Figure 4.9). This is a hereditary ectodermal dysplasia with thickening of the nails which become yellow-brown tubular, hard and barrel-shaped. They project upwards at their free edge while the subungual tissue is filled with keratotic material. The nail dystrophy usually appears within the first 6 months of life but later occurrence has been reported. Paronychia and onycholysis are common as well as recurrent shedding of the nail.

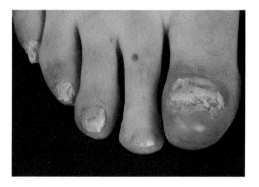

FIGURE 4.6
Lichen planus.

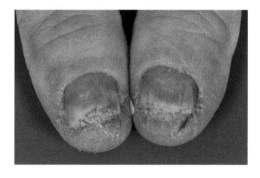

FIGURE 4.7
Contact dermatitis.

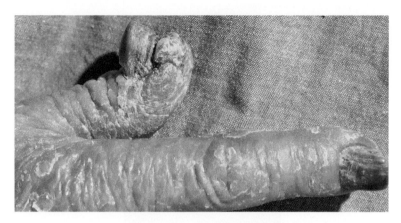

FIGURE 4.8
Erythroderma.

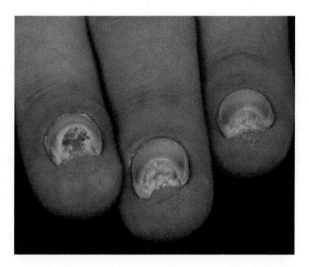

FIGURE 4.9
Pachyonychia congenita.

11. **Acrokeratosis paraneoplastica**. This occurs in association with malignancy of the upper respiratory or digestive tract. In severe forms, the free edge is raised by subungual hyperkeratosis. The lesions resemble advanced psoriatic nail dystrophy and may progress to complete loss of the diseased nails.

12. **Bowen's disease** (Figure 4.10). Classic patterns in periungual involvement include hyperkeratotic or papillomatous and even warty proliferation; erosions; scaling of the nail fold; whitish cuticle; periungual swelling from deep tumour proliferation; ulceration of the lateral nail groove is sometimes crusted with granulation-like tissue beneath the scab.

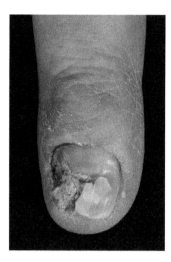

FIGURE 4.10
Bowen's disease.

4.2 Distal Lateral Subungual Onychomycosis with Marked Onycholysis

Onycholysis can appear in many different conditions (Figures 4.11–4.14, Table 4.1). In fingernails, primary onycholysis is frequently associated with secondary invasion by *Candida* and/or *Pseudomonas*. It should be differentiated from onycholysis due to overzealous cleaning with an orange stick, for example. Traumatic onycholysis of the toenails may present differently to that of fingernails. The diagnosis is obvious when the nail plate–nail bed separation appears after strenuous exercise in new footwear. Occasionally, a blackish hue may be the only presentation and is often due to the second toe overriding the big toe, which results in lateral subungual triangular haemorrhage. This is more common in women for obvious reasons [3]. Patients with the various forms of epidermolysis bullosa are more susceptible to onycholysis [4]. In Bowen's disease onycholysis is often associated with oozing erosion.

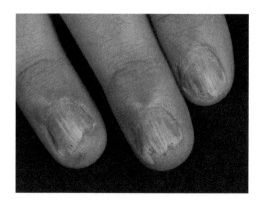

FIGURE 4.11
Lichen planus.

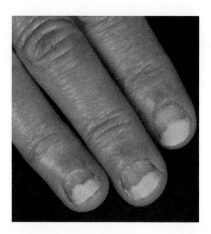

FIGURE 4.12
Onycholysis after manicure.

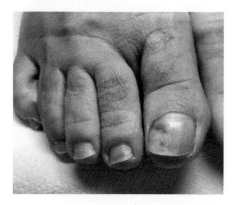

FIGURE 4.13
Traumatic onycholysis.

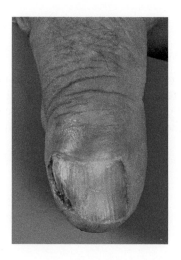

FIGURE 4.14
Bowen's disease.

TABLE 4.1

Differential Diagnosis of Fungal Onycholysis

Nail infection	Systemic conditions
Bacterial: *Pseudomonas, Proteus mirabilis* Viral: herpes simplex, warts	Acrokeratosis paraneoplastica Cancers Iron deficiency Lupus erythematosus, scleroderma
Dermatological disease	Pregnancy Raynaud's disease
Bullous diseases Contact dermatitis, atopic dermatitis Cutaneous T lymphoma Langerhans histiocytosis	Thyroidism Yellow nail syndrome
Lichen planus Pachyonychia congenita	**Congenital and/or hereditary disease**
Psoriasis/Reiter's syndrome Subungual tumours (benign or malignant)	Epidermolysis bullosa Hereditary partial onycholysis (Schulze)
Chemical causes	**Drugs**
Alkalis, mineral oils Cosmetics (depilatories) Detergents and solvents Hydrofluoric acid Sodium hypochlorite Sugar	Cytotoxics (bleomycin, 5-fluorouracil, docetaxel, paclitaxel, etc.) Etretinate, acitretin, isotretinoin Psoralens, cyclines, fluoroquinolones (responsible for photo-onycholysis)
Physical causes	
Burn Foreign body implantation Manicure Occupational factors Overlapping of the toes Repeated microtrauma Sport enthusiasts	

4.3 Superficial White Onychomycosis

Superficial friability can be produced by keratin granulations due to nail varnish or to base coat (Figure 4.15). Parakeratotic psoriatic cells, which usually disappear from the nail surface, leaving pitting, may be abnormally adherent to each other for a long period, producing white superficial patches. An identical presentation may be observed in alopecia areata.

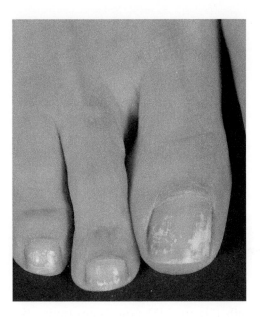

FIGURE 4.15
Keratin granulation.

4.4 Proximal Subungual White Onychomycosis without Paronychia

This type of fungal infection, which may present with varied features [5], can be mimicked by:

- Congenital leukonychia (Figure 4.16).
- Transverse leukonychia that may be monodactylous (single trauma, liquid nitrogen on the proximal nail fold or febrile infectious diseases and erythema multiforme),

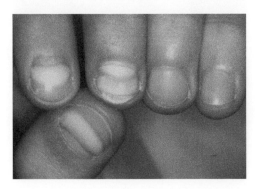

FIGURE 4.16
Congenital leukonychia.

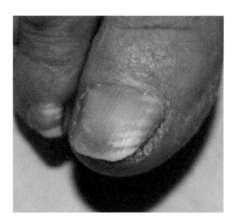

FIGURE 4.17
Traumatic transverse leukonychia due to poor fitting shoes.

or polydactylous (excessive manicure); it may also be due to repeated microtrauma to untrimmed toenails (Figure 4.17). Sometimes traumatic leukonychia can also present as punctata (Figure 4.18).

- Psoriatic transverse leukonychia is often accompanied by pitting of the nail and oil droplets.
- Neurological disorders such as sympathetic reflex dystrophy and spinal cord injury.

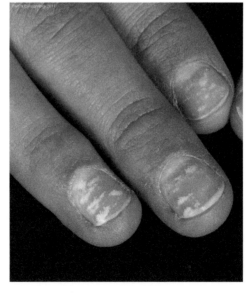

FIGURE 4.18
Traumatic punctate leukonychia.

TABLE 4.2

Main Causes of Chronic or Subacute Paronychia

Infective

- Bacterial
  - staphylococci, streptococci
  - *Pseudomonas, Proteus mirabilis*
  - syphilis
- Viral
  - herpes
  - warts (beneath the proximal nail fold)
- Parasitic (tungiasis)

Dermatological

- contact dermatitis
- parakeratosis pustulosa
- psoriasis, Reiter's syndrome
- in-growing toenail
- pemphigus
- Darier's disease

Drugs

- antiretroviral drugs
- cytotoxic drugs
- retinoids

Microtrauma

- Manicure

4.5 Proximal Subungual White Onychomycosis with paronychia

This type of fungal infection can be mimicked by any factor that causes paronychia with subsequent nail dystrophy (Table 4.2).

4.6 Fungal Melanonychia

Haematoma, subungual tumours, foreign bodies, longitudinal melanonychia and in particular malignant melanoma should be ruled out (Figures 4.19–4.23, Table 4.3). Dermoscopy examination of any blackish nail is the first step in reaching the proper diagnosis before excisional biopsy.

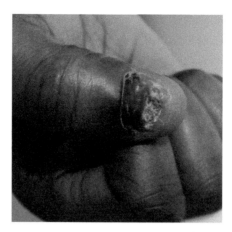

FIGURE 4.19
Fungal melanonychia due to *Trichophyton soudanense*.

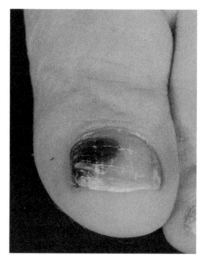

FIGURE 4.20
Fungal melanonychia due to *Trichophyton rubrum*.

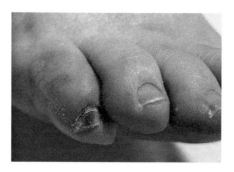

FIGURE 4.21
Frictional melanonychia.

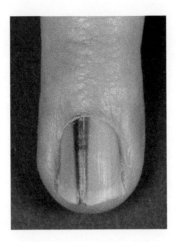

FIGURE 4.22
Acral melanoma.

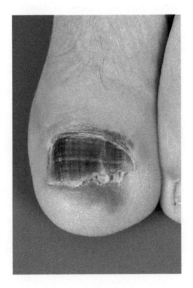

FIGURE 4.23
Melanoma with periungual hyperpigmentation (Hutchinson sign).

TABLE 4.3

Fungal Causes of Melanonychia (Some of These Fungi May Be Only Possible Causative Organisms) [6]

Acrothecium nigrum
Aureobasidium pullulans
Alternaria grisea
Candida albicans
Candida humicola
Candida tropicalis
Chaetomium globosum
Chaetomium kunze
Chaetomium perpulchrum
Cladophialophora carrionii
Cladosporium sphaerospermum
Curvularia lunata
Fusarium oxysporum
Hormodendrum elatum
Phyllosticta sydowii
Pyrenochaeta unguis-hominis
Scopulariopsis brumptii
Scytalidium dimidiatum (Nattrassia mangiferae, Hendersonula toruloidea)
Trichophyton mentagrophytes var. *Mentagrophytes*
Trichophyton rubrum
Trichophyton soudanense
Wangiella dermatitidis

References

1. Kyriakou A, Zagalioti SC, Trakatelli MG, et al. Fungal infections and nail psoriasis: an update. *J Fungi (Basel)*. 2022;8(2):154.
2. Lim SS, Chamberlain A, Hur K, et al. Dermoscopic evaluation of inflammatory nail disorders and their mimics. *Acta Derm Venereol*. 2021;101(9):adv00548.
3. Ramos Pinheiro R, Dias Domingues T, Sousa V, et al. A comparative study of onychomycosis and traumatic toenail onychodystrophy dermoscopic patterns. *J Eur Acad Dermatol Venereol*. 2019;33(4):786–92.
4. Baran R, Badillet G. Primary onycholysis of the big toenail: a review of 113 cases. *Br J Dermatol*. 1982;106:529–34.
5. Iorizzo M, Starace M, Pasch MC. Leukonychia: what can white nails tell us? *Am J Clin Dermatol*. 2022;23(2):177–93.
6. Starace M, Ambrogio F, Bruni F, et al. Dermatophytic melanonychia: a case series of an increasing disease. *Mycoses*. 2021 May;64(5):511–19.

5

Onychoscopy of Onychomycosis

Bianca Maria Piraccini and Luca Rapparini

5.1 Introduction

Onychoscopy (nail dermatoscopy) plays a key role in the diagnosis and differential diagnosis of most diseases of the nail apparatus, including onychomycosis, being an easy-to-perform, quick and non-invasive procedure. Although the definitive diagnosis of onychomycosis relies on mycology or histopathology, in poor settings where laboratory testing is not feasible, onychoscopy is a useful tool for the clinician [1,2].

Onychoscopy technique is more complex than dermatoscopy of the skin, due to the nail size, shape and hardness [3]. Dry dermatoscopy allows evaluation of the nail surface and is particularly useful in superficial onychomycosis, while using the gel as an interface is useful for studying nail colour changes and onycholysis [4,5]. In addition to being useful for diagnosis, onychoscopy is also useful as a guide to locating the best site to perform nail abrasion for microbiological samples [6].

5.2 Distal Subungual Onychomycosis (DSO)

5.2.1 Onychoscopy of Distal Subungual Onychomycosis (DSO)

Onychoscopy allows better observation of the three signs that characterize DSO, namely onycholysis, subungual hyperkeratosis and colour changes determined by the parasitation of the fungus at the stratum corneum level of the nail bed [1,4]. The involved nails should be examined both horizontally and frontally, as frontal observation allows the study of the distal margin and subungual space.

Specific onychoscopy features of DSO, mainly seen in the toenails, include [7,8]:

1. *Nail Plate/Nail Bed Detachment*: Onycholysis: It has an irregular, fringed, jagged proximal margin [4] (Figure 5.1).
2. *Subungual Hyperkeratosis:* The reactive hyperproliferation of the bed and the hyphae accumulate under the nail inducing the lifting of the nail plate. Subungual hyperkeratosis is better evaluated by looking at the nail frontally: the subungual scales have a typical irregular accumulation with a *ruin-like appearance* and are yellow-orange-white in colour (Figure 5.2) [2,9].

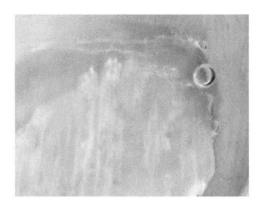

FIGURE 5.1
Onychoscopy of DSO showing a jagged proximal margin of the onycholysis.

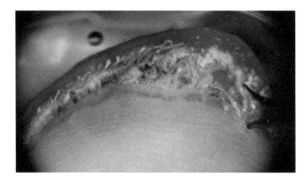

FIGURE 5.2
Onychoscopy of the distal nail margin in DSO: the nail plate is uplifted by multicoloured (yellow, white, orange) subungual scales with a *ruin-like appearance*.

3. *Colour Alterations:* The colour changes are due to fungus presence under and within the nail plate. Longitudinal striae, not always visible to the naked eye, can take on different colours, represented by white, yellow and orange. The onychoscopy finding of whitish-yellow longitudinal striae under the nail plate is characteristic and the fringed, *spikes* appearance is due to the hyphae which dig indentations along the bed in a disto-proximal direction (Figure 5.3) [7]. Presence of fungal colonies within the nail plate induces loss of transparency and the appearance of multiple focal homogeneous white patches, often associated with peripheral tiny cotton-like opacities, over and within the nail plate (Figure 5.4).

The diffuse opaque yellowish-orange colour of the nail is due to the detachment of the nail plate from the bed and the presence of hyphae and scales; the discoloration, fading in colour with a blurred pattern is called *aurora borealis pattern* [7]. When a brown-black colour is present, we are dealing with a variant of onychomycosis which takes the name of pigmented onychomycosis (see dedicated paragraph).

Nail plate invasion by hyphae causes its loss of transparency and therefore it no longer reflects the characteristic white-pink of the bed, becoming matte white.

Other nonspecific onychoscopy findings include an irregular distal margin, linked to the fact that the nail plate, following the fungal invasion, becomes more fragile and

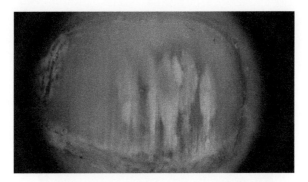

FIGURE 5.3
Onychoscopy of DSO: yellow-orange longitudinal striae with colour fading from orange to yellow to white.

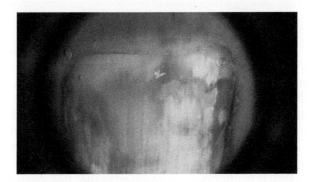

FIGURE 5.4
Onychoscopy of DSO: multiple focal homogeneous opaque white patches, with peripheral tiny cotton-like opacities.

fragmented, and subungual purple-black dots and globules, due to subungual haemorrhages [7].

Toenail DSO caused by dermatophytes is often associated with hyperkeratotic moccasin-type tinea pedis plantaris, which at the dermatoscopic level is characterized by a fine diffuse desquamation of the sole of the foot.

DSO caused by non-dermatophytic moulds (*Scopulariopsis brevicaulis, Fusarium* sp., *Acremonium* sp.) has the onychoscopic characteristics described above, but it is often possible to appreciate an important reddening of the periungual skin, linked by the quick marked inflammatory response of the host to the mould invasion.

Onychoscopy of fingernail DSO shows onycholysis and mild subungual hyperkeratosis. The nail plate is thin and therefore it is easily invaded by the fungus and becomes brittle and whitish.

DSO can also present with peculiar variants, such as dermatophytoma and pigmented onychomycosis, which are treated in a separate paragraph.

5.2.2 Differential Diagnosis

5.2.2.1 Nail Psoriasis

It is the main differential diagnosis of toenail DSO, and also the most difficult. When psoriasis is limited to the big toes, it can present with nonspecific features, such as onycholysis

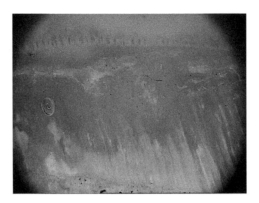

FIGURE 5.5
Onychoscopy of nail psoriasis showing a slightly dented proximal margin, surrounded by a bright yellow nail bed pigmentation.

and hyperkeratosis. Psoriasis onycholysis at onychoscopy shows a slightly dented proximal margin, the hyperkeratosis of the bed is characterized by tightly adherent white scales, not yellowish-white flaky, and the colour of the nail is bright yellow in a band that surrounds the onycholysis (Figure 5.5). It is also important to look for additional onychoscopic signs suggestive of psoriasis, such as salmon patches of the nail bed, which appear as round bright yellow patches under the transparent nail plate, and pitting, characterized by irregular shape, size and distribution of the pits [4]. In psoriasis, moreover, high-magnification dermoscopy of the hyponychium shows irregularly distributed, dilated, tortuous, elongated capillaries [10]. It is important to emphasize that nail psoriasis and onychomycosis may rarely be associated, so the onychoscopy characteristics of the two pathologies can be overlapping.

5.2.2.2 Traumatic Onycholysis

Traumatic onycholysis represents another important differential diagnosis of onychomycosis where onychoscopy can allow diagnosis. Traumatic onycholysis is characterized by a linear proximal edge of onycholysis and by a normally pale pink bed (Figure 5.6). Subungual hyperkeratosis is absent or white and less pronounced than DSO [3]. The specificity of the dermoscopy signs "jagged edge" and "longitudinal striae" in DSO is 100%, and the specificity and sensibility of the sign "linear edge" in traumatic onycholysis are 100% [7].

5.2.2.3 Acquired Pachyonychia/Onychogryphosis

Typical of the toenails of the elderly, the nail plate is thick and opaque so that it is not possible to observe below the plate with onychoscopy.

5.2.2.4 Onychomatricoma

It is a benign tumour of the nail matrix characterized by thickening of the affected nail plate with longitudinal yellow discoloration, transverse excessive curvature and splinter haemorrhages. Onychoscopy shows regular longitudinal white streaks that reach the distal margin, with splinter haemorrhages and elongated vessels within. An onychoscopy

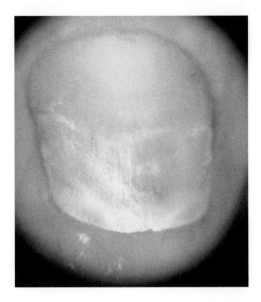

FIGURE 5.6
Onychoscopy of traumatic onycholysis showing a linear proximal edge of onycholysis and a normally pale pink bed.

of the distal margin of the nail allows the diagnosis as it shows the thickening of the yellowish part of the nail plate with multiple holes with a honeycomb appearance [9]. Onychomatricoma may be a predisposing factor for onychomycosis because the channels within the nail plate provide a favourable environment for fungal invasion [11].

5.2.2.5 Acute Bacterial Paronychia

It enters the differential diagnosis with onychomycosis caused by non-dermatophyte moulds: in both pathologies, dermoscopy of the periungual tissues shows significant inflammation, but in bacterial paronychia the nail plate appears healthy, unlike onychomycosis due to non-dermatophyte moulds where the onychoscopic characteristics typical of onychomycosis are found.

5.2.3 Onychoscopy of Dermatophytoma

Dermatophytoma is represented by an accumulation of hyphae and scales under the nail plate, which is difficult for antifungals to penetrate.

At the onycoscopic level, it appears as a round, irregular-shaped area of a homogeneous matte yellow-orange colour, below the plate, which continues distally with a yellow-whitish band of onycholysis (Figure 5.7) [12].

5.2.4 Onychoscopy of Pigmented Onychomycosis

It is caused by the melanoides variant of *Trichophyton rubrum* which produces melanin that is deposited among the scales. It clinically presents itself as melanonychia which can be misdiagnosed as melanoma. Onychoscopy allows the diagnosis as it shows that the black colour is associated with the other typical characteristics of DSO, with subungual scales

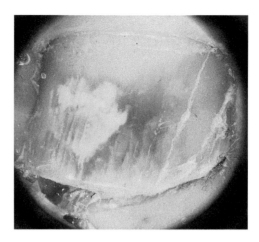

FIGURE 5.7
Onychoscopy of dermatophytoma: irregularly round opaque yellow-orange area below the nail plate, with multiple distal longitudinal striae reaching the distal margin.

with multicoloured pigmentation, which often organize themselves in longitudinal bands under the nail plate [4]. The distal margin shows accumulation of multicoloured scales (Figure 5.8).

Less frequently, melanonychia associated with onychomycosis is a true melanocytic pigmentation due to nail matrix melanocyte activation as a result of inflammation generated by onychomycosis [13].

5.2.5 Differential Diagnosis

In pigmented onychomycosis, onychoscopy plays a fundamental role in the differential diagnosis with other pigmentations, both of melanocytic origin and exogenous pigmentations.

The main pathologies with which it enters the differential diagnosis are as follows.

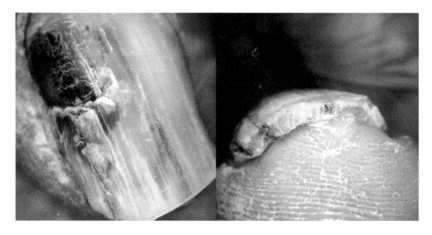

FIGURE 5.8
Onychoscopy of pigmented onychomycosis: multicoloured (black, yellow, orange) pigmentation of the nail plate and of the subungual scales.

5.2.5.1 *Subungual Hematoma*

A recent subungual hematoma appears as a red to black area with rounded edges, with "pseudopods" branching in the direction of the free edge [4], in contrast to DSO, in which the spikes are directed in the direction of the matrix. There is no subungual hyperkeratosis and does not reach the free edge of the nail [14].

5.2.5.2 *Melanonychia*

When faced with nail pigmentation, the first step is to determine whether or not the pigmentation is of melanocytic origin: in the latter case, a longitudinal band is generally observed at onychoscopy, more or less regular in shape, size, spacing, parallelism and colour, which affects the nail plate. The spikes and subungual hyperkeratosis typical of DSO are not present [15], and pigmentation localizes more to the distal lamina, rather than to the matrix/proximal lamina [2].

5.3 White Superficial Onychomycosis

In white superficial onychomycosis (WSO) the fungus directly invades the dorsal surface of the nail plate and descends towards the lower layers, feeding on hard keratins.

Onychoscopy features of WSO include white and yellow superficial scales. Initially it presents with white spots with a distinct edge which, due to coalescence, can progressively affect the entire nail, taking the name of trichophytic or mycotic leukonychia. The scales are better appreciated with dry dermatoscopy: the white flakes that are observed represent the colonies of *Trichophyton interdigitale* or, more rarely, some non-dermatophyte moulds. The whitish surface of the nail plate becomes rougher and softer, and long-standing lesions take on a more yellowish appearance (Figure 5.9) [16].

WSO can also present itself with a deep form, due to the non-dermatophytic moulds of *Acremonium* or *Fusarium*, where the nail plate is invaded throughout its depth [16]. At

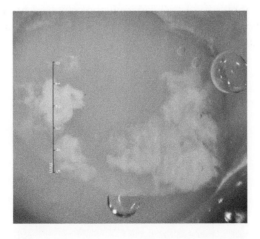

FIGURE 5.9
Onychoscopy of white superficial onychomycosis: non-homogeneous white, opaque and crumbly spots on the nail plate surface.

onychoscopy, it is characterized by white, opaque and crumbly spots that are localized not only on the surface, but also within the nail plate with surface irregularities. The patches merge with each other and begin to look not only white but also more yellowish because they reflect less light due to the massive deep deposition of the hyphae.

Superficial black onychomycosis caused by dematiaceous or black fungi shares the onychoscopic appearance of WSO, with the difference that in this case, the superficial scales are black [17].

5.3.1 Differential Diagnosis

5.3.1.1 Punctate Leukonychia

It is due to nail trauma at the matrix level which produces a nail plate that has foci of parakeratotic cells that do not reflect light and appear as white spots. At onychoscopy, the surface of the nail plate appears smooth, as these white spots are located inside it [18]. For differential diagnosis with WSO, it is helpful to observe the behaviour of the white pigmentation following the application of gel on the nail plate: if it is applied on a punctate leukonychia spot, the spots do not disappear, if instead it is applied on onychomycosis, the spots disappear or fade [4].

5.3.1.2 Superficial Fragility of the Nail Plate

It is linked to the degranulation of keratin due to the prolonged use of semi-permanent nail polishes which, in their removal, completely degranulate the superficial keratin leading to formation of white superficial spots that simulate a WSO. The history is necessary for the differential diagnosis; at onychoscopy in nail fragility, the scales are more regular and compact, compared to the WSO where they appear less adherent [4].

5.4 Proximal Subungual Onychomycosis (PSO)

Onychoscopy typically shows a whitish opaque spot covered by a transparent nail plate initially located at the level of the lunula, then spreading distally over time and taking on a yellowish colour (Figure 5.10) [19].

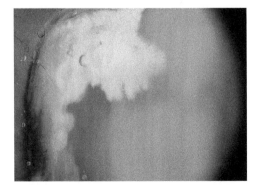

FIGURE 5.10
Onychoscopy of proximal subungual onychomycosis: whitish opaque irregular spot with fluffy margin involving the proximal nail.

5.4.1 Differential Diagnosis

5.4.1.1 Acute Bacterial Paronychia

It enters the differential diagnosis with PSO due to non-dermatophytic moulds, in which there is a great inflammation with the secretion of purulent material. At onychoscopy, the white-yellow discoloration in acute paronychia is within the proximal nail fold, being an abscess, and not under the nail plate.

5.5 Total Dystrophic Onychomycosis

Total dystrophic onychomycosis (TO) results from the evolution of all the types of onychomycoses described above, especially from a long-lasting DSO, but it can also be primary, above all in immunosuppressed subjects.

At onychoscopy, TO appears as an entirely opaque white or yellow thickened nail with a very brittle surface and distal margin. Since it crumbles easily, an abnormally thickened nail bed can be observed.

In the periungual tissues, hyperkeratotic areas can be found secondary to the invasion of dermatophytes in the surrounding tissues.

References

1. Gupta AK, Stec N, Summerbell RC, Shear NH, Piguet V, Tosti A, et al. Onychomycosis: a review. *J Eur Acad Dermatol Venereol*. 2020 Sep;34(9):1972–90.
2. Hazarika N, Chauhan P, Divyalakshmi C, Kansal NK, Bahurupi Y. Onychoscopy: a quick and effective tool for diagnosing onychomycosis in a resource-poor setting. *Acta Dermatovenerol Alp Pannon Adriat*. 2021 Mar;30(1): 11–14.
3. Piraccini BM, Bruni F, Starace M. Dermoscopy of non-skin cancer nail disorders: nail dermoscopy. *Dermatol Ther*. 2012 Nov;25(6):594–602.
4. Alessandrini A, Starace M, Piraccini BM. Dermoscopy in the evaluation of nail disorders. *Skin Appendage Disord*. 2017;3(2):70–82.
5. Hay RJ, Baran R. Onychomycosis: a proposed revision of the clinical classification. *J Am Acad Dermatol*. 2011 Dec;65(6):1219–27.
6. Bet DL, Reis ALD, Chiacchio ND, Belda Junior W. Dermoscopy and onychomycosis: guided nail abrasion for mycological samples. *An Bras Dermatol*. 2015 Dec;90(6):904–6.
7. Piraccini BM, Balestri R, Starace M, Rech G. Nail digital dermoscopy (Onychoscopy) in the diagnosis of onychomycosis: onychoscopy: digital dermoscope to diagnose onychomycosis. *J Eur Acad Dermatol Venereol*. 2013 Apr;27(4):509–13.
8. Piraccini B, Alessandrini A. Onychomycosis: a review. *J Fungi*. 2015 Mar 27;1(1):30–43.
9. Iorizzo M, Starace M, Di Altobrando A, Alessandrini A, Veneziano L, Piraccini BM. The value of dermoscopy of the nail plate free edge and hyponychium. *Acad Dermatol Venereol*. 2021 Dec;35(12):2361–6.
10. Iorizzo M, Dahdah M, Vincenzi C, Tosti A. Videodermoscopy of the hyponychium in nail bed psoriasis. *J Am Acad Dermatol*. 2008 Apr;58(4):714–15.
11. Kallis P, Tosti A. Onychomycosis and onychomatricoma. *Skin Appendage Disord*. 2015;1(4):209–12.

12. Lipner SR, Scher RK. Onychomycosis. *J Am Acad Dermatol*. 2019 Apr;80(4):835–51.
13. Cohen PR, Shurman J. Fungal melanonychia as a solitary black linear vertical nail plate streak: case report and literature review of candida-associated longitudinal melanonychia striata. *Cureus*. 2021 Apr 1;13(4):e14248.
14. Finch J, Arenas R, Baran R. Fungal melanonychia. *J Am Acad Dermatol*. 2012 May;66(5):830–41.
15. Piraccini BM, Dika E, Fanti PA. Tips for diagnosis and treatment of nail pigmentation with practical algorithm. *Dermatologic Clin*. 2015 Apr;33(2):185–95.
16. Piraccini BM, Tosti A. White superficial onychomycosis: epidemiological, clinical, and pathological study of 79 patients. *Arch Dermatol*. 2004;140(6):696–701.
17. Di Chiacchio N, Noriega LF, Gioia Di Chiacchio N, Ocampo-Garza J. Superficial black onychomycosis due to *Neoscytalidium dimidiatum*. *J Eur Acad Dermatol Venereol*. 2017 Oct;31(10):e453–5.
18. Iorizzo M, Starace M, Pasch MC. Leukonychia: what can white nails tell us? *Am J Clin Dermatol*. 2022 Mar;23(2):177–93.
19. Dompmartin D, Dompmartin A, Deluol AM, Grosshans E, Coulaud JP. Onychomycosis and AIDS: clinical and laboratory findings in 62 patients. *Int J Dermatol*. 1990 Jun;29(5):337–9.

6

Mycological Examination of the Nails

Pauline Lecerf and Bertrand Richert-Baran

6.1 Patient History

The patient's clinical medical history must first be collected, including any previous fungal infections, underlying health conditions and use of medications. This information is invaluable both for interpreting test results (such as culture, which may be negative under treatment) and before initiating treatment.

6.2 Clinical Examination

A careful examination should be performed to assess the number of fingers and/or toes affected, whether other sites are involved (e.g. *tinea pedis*, *cruris*) and to determine the clinical type of onychomycosis, to adapt the sampling technique and treatment accordingly.

6.3 Sampling

Nail sampling is mandatory to confirm the diagnosis and identify the pathogen. Antifungal treatments must be initiated only after mycological confirmation. It is imperative to take a high-quality mycological sample adapted to the type of onychomycosis.

All antifungal agents (topical and systemic) must be stopped 2–3 months before sampling (called the "wash-out time") [1].

Suspicious nails should be disinfected with 70% alcohol to remove contaminants from the environment (bacteria, yeasts, non-dermatophytic moulds).

One should cut as much as possible of the diseased nail plate to send a large amount of material to the lab and already downsize the fungal mass [2]. The infected nail plate must be cut as close as possible to the clinically healthy zone corresponding to the "mycelial front" (Figure 6.1a and b). This is where numerous alive hyphae are present, and it gives more chance to get a positive culture. Subungual debris must also be scraped and send to the lab; these are rich in filaments.

A large nail cutter (nail pliers or nipper for thick toenails), scalpel blade for scraping nail plate and a spoon excavator or any small blunt instrument (used in pedicure) can be

DOI: 10.1201/9781003381648-7

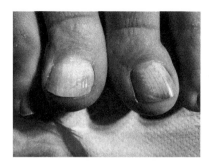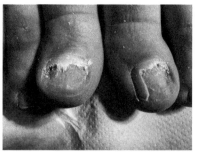

FIGURE 6.1
How to perform a correct sampling: remove as much as possible of infected keratin (debriding) and sample as close as possible to the proximal "mycelian front".

used for collection of subungual debris. These instruments may also be used in superficial onychomycosis to collect samples.

When a proximal subungual onychomycosis is suspected, a 3 mm (minimum) punch biopsy sample from the affected nail plate may be performed, taking care not to damage the underlying matrix. This requires a local block. Another option is to collect successive superficial chips with a 15 blade until reaching the deepest layer of the plate. This is totally painless.

Genuine nail biopsies (longitudinal nail biopsies or punch biopsies) encompassing not only the nail plate but also the dermis and the underneath epithelium are rarely performed to diagnose onychomycosis, except when another diagnosis, such as psoriasis or lichen planus, is clinically suspected.

Specimen is labelled indicating the history, clinical elements and the site of sampling (toe, finger). The samples are collected in a philatelic envelope or plastic boxes, depending on the laboratory rules in each country. One should note that it's better to not use plastic containers, such as sterile specimen jars, because the scales stick to the plastic (owing to static electricity).

6.4 Laboratory

6.4.1 Direct Microscopic Examination

Direct examination with potassium hydroxide (KOH) preparation and culture are the most employed tests. KOH mount is a simple, rapid and inexpensive test that requires minimal infrastructure, though some amount of experience is necessary to interpret the smears accurately.

For direct microscopy, the specimen is placed on a glass slide and covered with potassium hydroxide (KOH) 10%–20% solution or 0.025% Congo red (in 5% SDS) solution or with 20% tetraethyl ammonium hydroxide (TEAH) solution. Fluorescence optical staining increases the sensitivity of the microscopic preparation [1,3]. A coverslip is then placed on the specimen, and the slide is incubated in a moist chamber for 10–30 minutes. The KOH dissolves the host cellular material, exposing the fungal hyphae and spores for rapid identification under the light (or fluorescent) microscope. This simple technique is achievable in most laboratories of microbiology and could be performed in less than 2 hours.

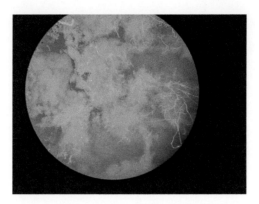

FIGURE 6.2
Direct examination of nail clipping in onychomycosis with Calcofluor. Note the branched filaments.

Examination is usually done at ×10 or ×20 magnification for branching hyphae, with confirmation using ×40 objective. Microscopic examination may also allow the detection of different morphological aspects which may help to specify the type of fungus involved, especially in onychomycosis (regular hyphae, sometimes dissociated in arthroconidia for dermatophytes [Figure 6.2]; irregular and poorly coloured or vesicular hyphae in a mould infection; blastoconidia associated or not to pseudohyphae in yeast infections). Dyes such as Congo red, Chicago blue, Parker ink, chlorazol black have been introduced onto KOH mounts allowing an easier visualization of fungal elements by phase contrast or fluorescence microscopy. While the sensitivity of KOH preparations is not very high, it can be increased by adding fluorescent brighteners (Calcofluor white). KOH can result in trapped air bubbles or fat droplets that lead to false-positive results as they resemble fungal structures [4].

6.4.2 Fungal Culture

The gold standard for mycological diagnosis is fungal culture. Dermatophytes grow in 2–6 weeks, depending on the species. This process allows the precise identification of the infecting agent but has a 30% false-negative rate. It requires the inoculation of the specimen onto a selective medium and examining for the morphological or microscopic features of colonies that develop after 10–21 days of incubation. Media used to culture dermatophytes (such as Sabouraud dextrose agar) typically contain antibiotics (gentamicin sulphate, chlortetracycline or chloramphenicol) and antifungals such as cycloheximide. These substances are useful in suppressing the growth of bacteria and moulds that would otherwise rapidly overgrow the more slowly growing dermatophytes [5–7].

Nail fragments should be placed onto the agar. Fungal cultures are stored at room temperature or usually incubated at 25°C±2°C (higher incubation temperatures of 30°C–32°C can be used if *Trichophyton verrucosum* infection is suspected). Cultures should be monitored and/or examined macro/microscopically once or twice weekly. The delay for optimal growth varies according to the species. They should be incubated for up to 30 days before declaring cultures to be negative, 6 weeks in case of suspected infections with *T. verrucosum*, *Trichophyton violaceum* or *Trichophyton soudanense*. The fungal colonies thus obtained are subsequently classified based on their macroscopic growth pattern, their colour as well as the formation of macroconidia and microconidia or other typical growth patterns as determined by microscopy (Figure 6.3). Sabouraud isolation medium, which contains

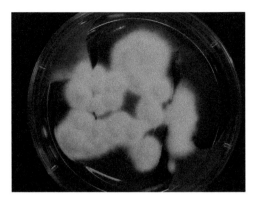

FIGURE 6.3
Culture of *Trichophyton rubrum* colonies.

dextrose, promotes mycelial growth, but sporulation may be lacking; so, when identification of dermatophyte isolates is not achievable directly from primary cultures, **subcultures** may be performed on specific media that stimulate both conidiation and the production of pigments. Cultural diagnosis demands the presence of an experienced staff capable of recognizing the subtle differential features of the colonies and to identify the fungus to the species level. The false-negative rate of fungal culture is ~40% or higher [8–10].

6.4.3 Histological Examination of the Nail Plate

In onychomycosis, histological examination is a microscopic examination of histological sections after staining of fungal polysaccharides to reveal the presence of fungi. Haematoxylin–eosin (H&E), Periodic acid–Schiff (PAS) and Grocott's methenamine stain (GMS) are used to visualize fungal elements and enhance hyphae by staining the fungal cell wall. It is a useful complementary technique, especially when there is strong clinical suspicion in the setting of a negative fungal culture and/or KOH preparation [7]. Histological examination in combination with fungal staining (PAS) or Grocott–Gomori staining can be recommended for previously treated patients with negative mycological test results. This laboratory method is the most sensitive procedure for the diagnosis of onychomycosis [3].

It allows visualization of the precise location of the invasive fungus inside the nail apparatus (Figure 6.4). The method also distinguishes various shapes of the fungal cells, in particular filamentous fungi, yeasts, conidia and sporodochia. PAS requires a specialized histology laboratory to process, embed, cut and stain the specimen as well as a trained pathologist to interpret it.

It only takes 2–7 days for results; however, its cost is significantly greater than that of a KOH preparation and culture. Histological analysis does not allow species identification. Alternate techniques have been used to determine the specific agent present in the histopathologic specimen, including immunohistochemistry, *in situ* hybridization, and polymerase chain reaction (PCR). Immunohistochemistry is a technique like histology. It is an upgraded technique where antibodies specific to the fungal pathogen are used to detect the causative organism. The labelled antibodies bind to the specific fungus and are detected by immunofluorescence, horseradish peroxidase enzyme or avidin–biotin complex. This diagnostic method is highly specific and eliminates false-positive contaminants.

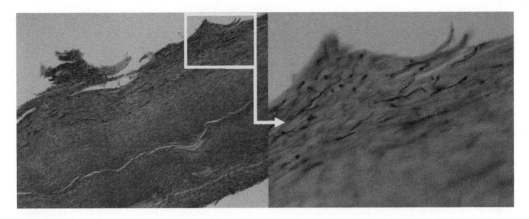

FIGURE 6.4
Histological examination of a superficial onychomycosis. Note the location of the filaments in the upper part of the plate.

Accurate diagnosis could be achieved by combining immunohistochemistry along with other techniques such as imaging to estimate the viability of the pathogen.

6.4.4 Molecular Methods for Pathogen Identification

With the advent of molecular diagnostics, identification of dermatophytes even to the strain level has been made easier, faster and more accurate. Molecular techniques are very sensitive and fast; they lead to results within days. Their specificity, however, is very heterogeneous. While culture diagnostics is a well-established procedure in most laboratories at present, the changeover to molecular biological techniques may require some effort. However, the investment strongly depends on which devices for PCR analyses or matrix-assisted laser desorption/ionization (MALDI)-time-of-flight mass spectrometry (TOF/MS) analyses are already in use and to what extent they can be utilized for dermatophyte diagnostics. In addition to the equipment purchase, the costs for consumables for molecular biological methods are higher than those for culture. In PCR, fluorescent labels or kits are expensive consumables. In contrast, however, the working time required for pathogen identification is much shorter [6].

6.4.4.1 Polymerase Chain Reaction and Quantitative PCR (qPCR)

In the last few years, direct pathogen detection at the DNA level from clinical material by PCR methods has become increasingly important. PCR for direct dermatophyte detection from skin scales and nail material is markedly more sensitive compared to fungal detection by culture [1,11].

Polymerase chain reaction (PCR) is a relatively simple and widely used molecular biology technique to amplify and detect DNA and RNA sequences. Compared to traditional methods of DNA cloning and amplification, which can often take days, PCR requires only a few hours. It is used to make multiple copies of a specific section of DNA. It allows thus to create a large amount of DNA from a small amount of DNA. Before performing a PCR, a specific DNA sequence of the pathogen must be extracted from the sample (clinical sample or dermatophyte culture). This is a preparation step before the PCR process. The effort required for DNA extraction prior to PCR varies from kit to kit. Some kits contain reagents for DNA extraction; others recommend the use of DNA extraction kits. The most frequently recommended kit is the QIAamp® DNA Mini Kit (Qiagen GmbH, Hilden) with an extended (90 minutes to 12 hours) initial lysis step. The Dermatophyte Kit from Statens Serum Institute and the DermaGenius® 2.0 kit each contains a two-buffer system for DNA extraction that requires only 10 minutes of incubation. PCR identifies fungal pathogens using specific dermatophyte primers. For the detection and differentiation of pathogenic fungi, a common target is the ribosomal genes, such as 18S rDNA, especially the so-called internal transcribed spacers ITS2 and ITS1. Besides ITS, the genes encoding chitinase-1 (CHS1), topoisomerase-2 (TOP2), β-tubulin (BTU) or translation elongation factor 1-α (EF-1-α) are also used. In contrast to other pathogenic fungi, dermatophyte species have a very high degree of phylogenetic similarity. The more variable ITS region is suitable for the differentiation of all known dermatophyte species, even if some differ only by one or two single-nucleotide polymorphisms (SNPs).

Real-Time PCR (RT-PCR) or quantitative PCR (qPCR) is a quantitative, sensitive technique. It is very similar to PCR, but it also allows to quantify the amount of target DNA present in a sample. Real-time PCR methods allow detection during the PCR reaction without the need for post-PCR steps. qPCR involves adding fluorescent dyes or probes that bind to the target DNA during amplification. These probes emit light at different wavelengths when they are excited by a laser. By measuring the light emitted at each wavelength, it can determine how much target DNA was present in the sample before amplification began. This way, the amplification of the DNA can be monitored in real time. RT-PCR takes longer than standard PCR, requires expensive laboratory equipment and trained personnel, and is not often used in a clinical setting.

PCR methods are more sensitive and significantly more rapid (24–48 hours versus 2–6 weeks for culture-based methods) than KOH microscopy and fungal culture and they have no problems in detecting pathogens that are growth inhibited by antimycotic therapy.

PCR methods have some limitations. They don't provide information regarding the viability of the organism and have high false-positive rates due to the potential identification of a contaminant. Moreover, this equipment is not available in all mycology labs and is expensive [1,8,9].

6.4.4.2 Matrix-Assisted Laser Desorption/Ionization Time-of-Flight Mass spectrometry (MALDI-TOF MS)

MALDI-TOF MS consists in preparing a biological sample, covering it with a so-called matrix, introducing it into a mass spectrometer, ionizing the molecules and measuring the time that each molecule takes to cover the distance between the origin and the detector. The result is a spectrum that can be compared to a database of spectra, whether it is a "homemade" or marketed database [10].

Prior to performing a MALDI-TOF MS, the biological sample must be prepared following different steps. Mass spectrometry requires a culture step. The protein must be extracted from the mycelium after dermatophyte culture. The most used medium is Sabouraud chloramphenicol-gentamicin (solid plate), with or without cycloheximide. Samples taken from the cultures must be free from any agar, as this later can negatively impact the identification. This culture medium is covered with a membrane intended to facilitate the recovery of the fungal colony for identification by mass spectrometry. After scraping the colonies, the next step is protein extraction. When the sample preparation is done, it is put on a MALDI-TOF MS target. This is called a spot. The manufacturer typically recommends a single spot for bacterial identification, some authors have advocated the use of several spots of the same sample to identify moulds and dermatophytes [10,12,13]. On the top of the spot (sample put on the target), a matrix is placed. The different MALDI-TOF systems available operate following different algorithms, either for the treatment of the raw spectra or for the identification processes, leading to differences in the identification scoring. The Maldi Biotyper software, associated with Bruker devices, preprocesses the raw spectrum and converts it into a mass list and the corresponding intensities. The mass list is then compared to the mass list of each reference spectra in the database.

Due to the high degree of phylogenetic similarity, the differentiation of dermatophyte species is challenging. For some closely related species, the differences in mass spectra have been reported to be insufficient or misleading, while for some other species they are too heterogeneous.

In contrast to bacteria and yeasts, commercial databases are poorly developed for identification of filamentous fungi, especially for identification of dermatophytes, and it led many teams to build "in-house" databases or to supplement commercial databases with homemade reference spectra. Most studies used homemade databases to enhance their correct identification rates [12,14,15].

Compared with conventional morphology-based techniques, MALDI-TOF is relatively inexpensive (per-unit identification), involves a rapid result turnaround time and yields more accurate results without the need for highly qualified staff. But progress is still needed at all steps of the process from culture to final analysis of the digital data [13].

6.4.4.3 Flow Cytometry

Flow cytometry is a molecular biology technique which relies on granularity, cell size, proteins and DNA markers, and generates distinct profiles of fungi to identify the pathogen. The fungal mass is collected from the specimen unit after treating with Tween 40 (a non-ionic detergent). It is then sorted by a dual flow cytometer according to its size based on staining fungal DNA with propidium iodide (PI) and fungal protein with fluorescein isothiocyanate (FITC), which aids in distinguishing fungi. However, this technique requires large sample sizes to identify the causative organism and is expensive due to its specialized equipment and requirement of trained staff [16].

References

1. Nenoff P, Reinel D, Mayser P, Abeck D, Bezold G, Bosshard PP, et al. S1 Guideline onychomycosis. *JDDG J Dtsch Dermatol Ges.* 2023;21(6):678–92.
2. Lecerf P, André J, Richert B. Prise en charge des onychomycoses. *Presse Méd.* Nov 2014;43(11):1240–50.
3. Lecerf P, Abdy S, Vollono L, Pastushenko I, Richert B, André J. Direct examination, histopathology and fungal culture for the diagnosis of onychomycosis: a retrospective, comparative study on 2245 specimens. *Mycoses.* févr 2021;64(2):187–93.
4. Velasquez-Agudelo V, Cardona-Arias JA. Meta-analysis of the utility of culture, biopsy, and direct KOH examination for the diagnosis of onychomycosis. *BMC Infect Dis.* 2017;17(1):166. Disponible sur: https://www.ncbi.nlm.nih.gov/pmc/articles/PMC5320683/

5. Robert R, Pihet M. Conventional methods for the diagnosis of dermatophytosis. *Mycopathologia*. déc 2008;166(5–6):295–306. Disponible sur: https://pubmed.ncbi.nlm.nih.gov/18478359/

6. Gümral R, Döğen A, Ilkit MM. Comparison of the contamination rates of culture media used for isolation and identification of dermatophytes. *Turk J Med Sci*. 2015;45(3):587–92.

7. Summerbell RC, Cooper E, Bunn U, Jamieson F, Gupta AK. Onychomycosis: a critical study of techniques and criteria for confirming the etiologic significance of nondermatophytes. *Med Mycol*. févr 2005;43(1):39–59.

8. Gupta AK, Zaman M, Singh J. Fast and sensitive detection of *Trichophyton rubrum* DNA from the nail samples of patients with onychomycosis by a double-round polymerase chain reaction-based assay. *Br J Dermatol*. Oct 2007;157(4):698–703.

9. Elewski BE. Onychomycosis: pathogenesis, diagnosis, and management. *Clin Microbiol Rev*. juill 1998;11(3):415–29.

10. Packeu A, De Bel A, l'Ollivier C, Ranque S, Detandt M, Hendrickx M. Fast and accurate identification of dermatophytes by matrix-assisted laser desorption ionization-time of flight mass spectrometry: validation in the clinical laboratory. *J Clin Microbiol*. Sept 2014;52(9):3440–3.

11. Cuchí-Burgos E, Rubio-Casino R, Ballestero-Téllez M, Pariente-Jiménez F, Pérez-Jové J, Blanco-Suárez A. Commercial real time PCR implementation for rapid diagnosis of onychomycosis: a new workflow in a clinical laboratory. *Enferm Infecc Microbiol Clín*. 1 août 2021;39(7):326–9.

12. Normand AC, Cassagne C, Gautier M, Becker P, Ranque S, Hendrickx M, Piarroux R. Decision criteria for MALDI-TOF MS-based identification of filamentous fungi using commercial and in-house reference databases. *BMC Microbiol*. 2017;17(1):25. Disponible sur: https://www.ncbi.nlm.nih.gov/pmc/articles/PMC5282874/

13. Normand AC, Cassagne C, Ranque S, L'Ollivier C, Fourquet P, Roesems S, et al. Assessment of various parameters to improve MALDI-TOF MS reference spectra libraries constructed for the routine identification of filamentous fungi. *BMC Microbiol*. 8 avr 2013;13:76.

14. Calderaro A, Motta F, Montecchini S, Gorrini C, Piccolo G, Piergianni M, et al. Identification of dermatophyte species after implementation of the in-house MALDI-TOF MS database. *Int J Mol Sci*. 11 Sept 2014;15(9):16012–24.

15. Lecerf P, De Paepe R, Jazaeri Y, Normand AC, Martiny D, Packeu A. Evaluation of a liquid media MALDI-TOF MS protocol for the identification of dermatophytes isolated from tinea capitis infections. *J Fungi Basel Switz*. 26 Nov 2022;8(12):1248.

16. Arrese JE, Piérard-Franchimont C, Greimers R, Piérard GE. Fungi in onychomycosis. A study by immunohistochemistry and dual flow cytometry. *J Eur Acad Dermatol Venereol*. 1 avr 1995;4(2):123–30.

7

Goals for the Treatment of Onychomycosis

Vishal Gaurav and Chander Grover

7.1 Introduction

Onychomycosis, or fungal nail infection, is a prevalent mycotic condition that affects a substantial proportion of the global population. It is caused by dermatophytes, yeasts and non-dermatophyte moulds (NDMs). Managing onychomycosis is challenging due to the slow nail growth rate and the difficulty in achieving sustained drug delivery at the site of infection [1]. However, advancements in antifungal therapy have paved the way for better drug penetration and more successful treatment outcomes.

As we embark on the long journey to treat onychomycosis, it is relevant and pertinent to define the goals for therapy. Physician and patient expectations regarding the outcome of treatment are shaped by diverse perspectives on what constitutes a cure (Table 7.1) [2]. However, physicians frequently neglect the communication regarding probable treatment outcomes to their patients. Existing data from onychomycosis treatment trials also pose challenges in interpretation and comparison as multiple definitions of "cure" exist and various measures are used to evaluate treatment effectiveness. While treating onychomycosis, the primary aim is eradication of the fungal pathogen from the affected nail, better understood as "mycological cure". However, an equally important aim is restoration of the appearance and functionality of affected nail, defined as "clinical cure". Published studies report various combinations and interpretations of mycological cure (typically defined as negative potassium hydroxide [KOH] microscopy and culture outcomes), clinical cure (typically defined as a percentage [e.g. 80%–100%] of visibly infection-free nail plate) or complete cure (combination of mycological and clinical cure) to establish efficacy and define cure (Table 7.2) [3–5].

This chapter explores the therapeutic goals for managing onychomycosis which should be kept in mind while deciding a treatment plan. These include an eradication of the fungal infection, prevention of recurrence and community spread, enhancement of appearance of the affected nails, improvement in patient's quality of life and prevention of development of antifungal resistance. These are detailed below.

7.2 Eradication of Fungal Infection

The main goal in the treatment of onychomycosis is to completely eliminate the fungal infection. There are various treatment options available, including topical therapies,

DOI: 10.1201/9781003381648-8

TABLE 7.1

Criteria for Determining Cure and Non-cure in Patients with Onychomycosis (See Further Ref. 2)

	Cure	Non-cure
EITHER	Complete absence of observable signs of onychomycosis (no need for mycological examination)	Positive mycological results
OR	Negative results from mycological laboratory tests, with one or more of the following two clinical signs: • Distal subungual hyperkeratosis or onycholysis affecting less than 10% of the nail plate • Thickening of the nail plate due to a concurrent medical condition that remains unchanged despite antifungal treatment	Negative mycological results, but with any of the following four clinical signs: • Persistent significant alterations (over 10%) in the nail plate indicative of dermatophyte infection • Appearance of white/yellow or orange/brown patches or streaks on/beneath the nail • Lateral onycholysis accompanied by debris within an otherwise clear nail plate • Hyperkeratosis on the lateral edge of the nail plate or nailfold

TABLE 7.2

Various Definitions Used for Evaluating Treatment Efficacy in Onychomycosis [3–5]

Treatment Goals	Definition
Mycological cure	Negative microscopy and culture (on two consecutive occasions, 4 weeks apart)
Clinical cure	Complete absence of all lesions on each nail (based on sequential photographs)
Complete cure	Both mycological and clinical cure
Almost complete cure	≤5% clinical involvement and mycological cure
Clinical success	<10% affected nail compared to baseline, with normalized nail growth
Clinical improvement	Reduction in total affected nail area which is >20% compared to baseline

systemic antifungals and physical or device-based methods including laser therapy (Table 7.3) [6]. A successful treatment approach should specifically target the underlying pathogen, eradicating it from the affected nail and the surrounding tissues. The choice of treatment depends on several factors such as the severity of infection, patient characteristics and medical history.

The evaluation of treatment effectiveness requires a comprehensive understanding of two fundamental concepts: mycological cure and clinical cure. Mycological cure refers to the complete eradication of the fungal pathogen from the nail plate and the surrounding tissues. On the other hand, clinical cure involves the resolution of visible symptoms and the restoration of the nail's normal appearance. Both types of cure play a significant role in assessing treatment outcomes, determining the evaluation methods used and understanding how these concepts interact in clinical practice. Having a clear understanding of these concepts is essential for optimal patient management and ensuring long-term treatment success [7].

TABLE 7.3

Treatment Options for Onychomycosis

Treatment Approach	Treatment Options
Topical antifungals	Amorolfine, ciclopirox, efinaconazole, tavaborole, etc.
Oral antifungals	Terbinafine, itraconazole, fluconazole, etc.
Lasers and other energy-based devices	Nd:YAG, fractional CO_2, dual-diode, near infrared, PDT, etc.
Surgical approach	Surgical removal or debridement, chemical debridement, mechanical abrasion, etc.

7.2.1 Mycological Cure

Mycological cure is considered the gold standard for evaluating treatment success and helps prevent recurrence of the infection. It refers to the complete elimination of the fungal pathogen from the nail and surrounding tissues. It can be determined by various laboratory techniques including direct microscopy, culture and molecular tests, which aid in identifying the causative organism, determining susceptibility to antifungals and monitoring treatment response [1,8]. Gupta et al. [9] used mycological cure as the outcome measure for comparison between three groups of patients with toenail onychomycosis. Group I received terbinafine 250 mg/day for 4 weeks, followed by 4 weeks off, and then an additional 4 weeks. Group II received terbinafine 250 mg/day for 12 weeks. Group III received itraconazole with a pulse of 400 mg/day for 7 days on and 21 days off, repeated three times. The mycological cure rates were 83.7%, 78.1% and 56.7% for Group I, Group II and Group III, respectively ($P=0.01$ for Group I vs. III). The study concluded that the intermittent terbinafine regimen provided similar efficacy and safety as the continuous terbinafine regimen and better effective cure rates compared to pulse itraconazole therapy [9].

As per strict criteria, mycological cure requires both negative culture and negative direct microscopy, whereas less rigid criteria consider only negative culture results, not taking direct microscopy into account. Disparities in the outcomes of various studies depend on the use of strict vs. less rigid criteria. The less rigid criteria are based on the fact that standard light microscopy cannot distinguish between dead and live hyphae; hence, their presence cannot be conclusively interpreted as an active fungal infection. However, relying solely on negative culture for defining cure is also inaccurate as the presence of a fungal isolate from a normal nail does not indicate an infection. Similarly, an abnormal nail lacking mycological confirmation does not rule out fungal infection. Many a times, successful elimination of the fungus may still be associated with residual abnormalities entirely unrelated to the infection (e.g. onychoschizia) or caused by long-standing damage due to disease (e.g. onycholysis) [10].

7.2.2 Clinical Cure

It focuses on resolution of visible signs and symptoms of onychomycosis, including nail discoloration, thickening, crumbling and subungual debris. Assessing clinical cure involves subjective observations and objective measurements, including nail appearance assessment, patient self-reporting and clinician evaluation [2,10]. Yadav et al. [11] used clinical cure for comparing treatment results between continuous terbinafine 250 mg daily for 12 weeks and three pulses of terbinafine (each of 500 mg daily for a week) repeated every 4 weeks. The clinical cure rates were 86.8% and 71.1% for the two groups, respectively

(P=0.280), while mycological cure rates were 28.9% and 18.4%, respectively (P=0.280). The study concluded that terbinafine pulse dosing was as effective as continuous dosing in treating onychomycosis [11].

Clinical cure is crucial for patients' satisfaction, as it directly affects their quality of life, self-esteem and social interactions. However, relying solely on it should be avoided, and both patients and physicians should maintain realistic expectations as nail appearance can be influenced by various internal and external factors. Injury to the nail unit, especially the nail bed and plate, may have occurred prior to the onset of onychomycosis, and even with mycological negativity, the restoration of a visually normal nail may not occur. Even with mycological cure, up to 10% of the nail surface may retain an abnormal appearance. At the same time, with clinical cure, mycological assessments are not necessary. However, some physicians view mycological confirmation as the preferred practice [2,10].

The OSI (Onychomycosis Severity Index) is a straightforward clinical scale assessing various parameters of involvement such as the percentage of nail plate affected, proximity of infection to the nail matrix, degree of subungual hyperkeratosis and presence of a dermatophytoma (Table 7.4). The inter-observer reliability of the OSI was found to be high among dermatology experts specializing in nail diseases, as well as dermatologists without specific expertise in nail diseases observing both photographed and live nails, making it an easy-to-learn and consistent tool. In general, a nail with a low OSI score is more likely to respond to conventional therapy, while high OSI score would pose greater challenges in treatment. Overall, nails with moderate involvement scored as 6 would be comparatively easier to treat than those scored as 15, and severe nail involvement scored as 16 would be relatively easier to treat than the ones scored as 35 [12].

7.2.3 Complete Cure

Complete cure refers to the successful and permanent elimination of the fungal infection, resulting in the restoration of a healthy and normal nail. This is the ultimate objective in treating onychomycosis, as it ensures complete eradication of the fungal pathogen and prevents any recurrence or further spread of the infection. It is characterized by the absence of any clinical involvement in the target nail and achievement of mycologic cure [2,10].

7.2.4 Target Nail for Evaluating Cure

While assessing cure, the primary focus is often on the great toenail, which serves as the designated target nail in most studies. It determines the overall success of the tested systemic antifungal drugs in clinical trials. This means that physicians typically rely on data specifically related to the great toe nail, while often disregarding other affected toenails.

The selection of the great toenail as target nail is based on its suitability to enable accurate measurement of the areas affected by the infection in comparison to healthy nail areas. Due to its larger size, it facilitates easier and more precise calculations. However, there are potential drawbacks of considering it solely, without taking into account the other toenails. It is susceptible to various forms of trauma, particularly repetitive minor trauma, which can in turn lead to permanent nail deformities. Research suggests that complete cure rates for the great toenail tend to be lower as compared to the second, third and fourth toenails. The second toenail, in particular, demonstrates the most favourable clinical outcomes based on the study results [10].

TABLE 7.4

Severity Evaluation of Onychomycosis with Onychomycosis Severity Index

Affected Nail (%)	Score
Area of Involvement[a]	
0	0
1–10	1
11–25	2
26–50	3
51–75	4
76–100	5

Proximity of Disease to Matrix

Extent of Involvement (Measured from Distal Free Edge)	Score
<¼	1
¼–½	2
½–¾	3
>¾	4
Matrix involvement	5

Dermatophytoma or Subungual Hyperkeratosis >2 mm

No	0
Yes	10

OSI = (Area score × Score for the proximity of disease to matrix) + 10 (if Yes)

Grading of Severity

0	Clinical cure
1–5	Mild onychomycosis
6–15	Moderate onychomycosis
16–35	Severe onychomycosis

[a] Measured using the boundaries of the lateral and proximal nail folds and distal nail groove. In cases with long-term onycholysis, the distal groove is used as an approximation for determining the area of involvement. If the affected nail has been trimmed by the patient or physician, an approximation of the area of involvement is done from the distal groove.

7.2.5 Real-World Interplay between These Factors

Although mycological and clinical cure are interrelated, they are not always in perfect alignment. In certain cases, patients may attain a mycological cure, effectively eliminating the fungus, but still experience clinical signs due to irreversible nail damage or slow nail regrowth. With topical antifungals, the mycological cure rates range from 10% to 30%, while clinical cure rates range from 10% to 40%. For systemic antifungals, the mycological cure rates tend to be higher (50%–70%), while clinical cure rates range from 50% to 80%. Achieving a complete cure can be more challenging and these rates with either topical or systemic antifungal treatments range from 5% to 30% [5]. As a result, it is crucial to adopt a comprehensive approach taking into account both mycological and clinical factors, the goal being to ensure a thorough assessment of treatment outcomes and minimize the risk of relapse [5]. Warshaw et al. (2001) compared three treatment groups receiving continuous terbinafine (250 mg/day), weekly intermittent terbinafine (500 mg/day for 1 week per month) and single monthly dose of terbinafine (1,000 mg/month), respectively. The complete cure rates were 20%, 40% and 0%; while mycological cure rates were 40%, 60% and 0% in the respective groups. The study highlights the wide differences between these cure rates [13].

Cure rates can vary depending on factors like severity of the infection, patient character-istics, treatment duration and compliance. Combination approaches, such as using topical antifungals for maintenance therapy following systemic treatment, may be considered to improve treatment outcomes and reduce the risk of recurrence [2,10].

Though clinical studies generally assess treatment success by focusing on the improve-ment of a single target toenail, in real-world scenarios, both patients and physicians con-sider the potentially varied responses of all nails. Although achieving mycological cure in a target toenail often aligns with similar patterns in the other nails, there are instances where one or more of the other toenails may continue to exhibit signs of infection. By combining systemic or topical antifungal medications with additional measures like nail debridement and patient education, the chances of treatment success are increased, and the likelihood of a relapse occurring is reduced. This holistic approach ensures compre-hensive treatment that addresses both the eradication of the fungal infection and the reso-lution of signs. However, it is crucial for patients to comprehend the difference between a cure and the visible appearance of treated nails, as there may be some residual changes following a prolonged infection [2,10].

7.3 Prevention of Recurrence

Even after a mycological cure, complete and permanent eradication of the infection may not be guaranteed. Recurrence of onychomycosis poses a frequent hurdle in effective man-agement. Hence, one of the key goals of treatment should be to prevent recurrence. Various useful preventive strategies include providing thorough patient education, promoting proper foot and nail hygiene, reducing exposure to environments with a high risk of rein-fection and implementing suitable preventive measures. These aim to safeguard against recurrence and maintain long-term treatment success [14,15].

7.3.1 Patient Education

Providing education to patients regarding onychomycosis, its risk factors and preventive measures plays a vital role in ensuring long-term success. It is crucial to inform patients about the significance of maintaining proper foot hygiene, regularly trimming their nails and refraining from sharing personal items. By highlighting the importance of early detection and timely treatment of fungal infections, the spread of onychomycosis to other nails or individuals can be prevented. By emphasizing these key points, patients can be empowered to take proactive steps in managing and preventing recurrence of their ony-chomycosis [15,16].

   a. *Foot and Nail Hygiene*: Maintaining proper foot and nail hygiene is vital to prevent any recurrence or reinfection. Patients should be counselled about the importance of keeping their feet clean and dry, opting for breathable footwear and regularly changing socks.
   b. *Proper Nail Trimming*: These techniques, avoiding injury or trauma to the nails, keep the nails at a short length to reduce the risk of fungal invasion.
   c. *Use of Antifungal Powders or Sprays*: These can be used in shoes and socks to play a role in preventing the recurrence of the infection.

By following these hygiene practices and incorporating preventive measures, patients can actively contribute to minimizing the chances of reinfection.

7.3.2 Preventive Measures

For individuals who have a history of recurrent onychomycosis or are particularly prone to fungal infections, implementing preventive measures becomes crucial. Options like topical antifungal therapy or intermittent systemic treatment may be taken into consideration. Prophylactic use of antifungal agents can be important in preserving a state free from fungal infection and decreasing the risk of reinfection [17].

After successful treatment, there is a higher likelihood of recurrence within the initial 2 years in approximately 20%–25% of cases. Overall recurrence rates range from 10% to 53%. The recurrence rates with itraconazole and terbinafine have been reported as 33.7% and 11.9%, respectively [5]. This recurrence can occur either as a relapse or a reinfection. Recurrences demonstrate a genetic predisposition and are more frequently observed in susceptible populations. The formation of fungal biofilms plays a significant role as it enhances resistance to treatment by creating an extracellular matrix (ECM) that shields the fungus, thereby establishing a reservoir of infection [18]. Using a topical antifungal solution twice a week can be effective for prophylaxis in treated cases. Prophylactic treatment with amorolfine lacquer, applied once every 2 weeks for a period of 3 years, has been shown to decrease the likelihood of recurrence [19]. Similarly, there is a potential benefit for maintenance treatment using efinaconazole. However, it is important to note that the risk–benefit profile of such treatment is currently unknown. Since efinaconazole is a topical solution, its systemic absorption is minimal, reducing the chances of drug interactions and acute liver injury [20,21].

7.3.3 Preventing Community Spread

Onychomycosis can spread within communities if proper preventive measures are not taken. Preventing spread to close contacts and to the community at large should be figured in while planning treatment of onychomycosis as it is an important goal of therapy. The following measures can be helpful for individuals.

a. *Minimizing Exposure to High-Risk Environments*: Specific environments can elevate the likelihood of spread of fungal infections. Public facilities such as swimming pools, saunas and communal showers tend to harbour fungi, making them particularly susceptible areas for infection. It is crucial to advise patients to wear protective footwear in these environments and thoroughly dry their feet after exposure. This can help reduce the risk of spread as well as the chances of fungal recurrence, maintaining long-term treatment success [21].

b. *Wearing Appropriate Footwear*: Well-fitting shoes that allow one's feet to breathe should be used. Occlusive footwear is a known risk factor. Socks made from breathable materials, such as cotton or moisture-wicking fabrics, should be preferred. Wearing damp or sweaty socks for extended periods should be avoided as this creates a favourable environment for fungal growth [17,21].

c. *Protection of Feet in Public Areas*: Shower shoes, sandals or flip-flops should be used in public places like swimming pools, gyms and communal showers. This helps prevent direct contact between feet and surfaces, reducing the risk of contamination [17,21].

d. *Avoid Sharing Personal Items*: One should refrain from sharing items like socks, shoes, nail clippers and towels with others. Fungal spores can survive on these items and transfer the infection from one person to another [17,21].

e. *Be Cautious at Nail Salons*: If visiting a nail salon, one should ensure that they follow strict hygiene practices. It should be made sure that the salon disinfects their tools properly, and uses clean, sterilized equipment for each customer. One can consider bringing own nail care tools if possible [17,21].

f. *Treating Existing Infections Promptly*: Early diagnosis and treatment are crucial for preventing the spread of infection to others [17,21].

7.4 Restoration of Nail Aesthetics and Functionality

Onychomycosis-induced nail deformities can lead to substantial psychological distress and have a detrimental effect on the patient's overall quality of life. Attaining a satisfactory cosmetic result is an essential goal in the comprehensive management of onychomycosis. In addition to eliminating the fungal infection, the treatment of onychomycosis should strive to enhance the appearance of the affected nail and restore functionality expected of it. By addressing the visible changes and restoring the nail's normal appearance, treatment aims to improve not only the physical aspects but also the psychological well-being of the patient. Various measures which can be helpful in this regard are detailed below.

7.4.1 Nail Debridement

Nail debridement is beneficial in several ways. It reduces the fungal load, particularly in cases such as dermatophytoma, where there is a concentrated fungal mass in the subungual area. It aids penetration by antifungal drugs, allowing them to reach the affected areas more effectively. It helps overcome challenges posed by biofilms and architectural abnormalities that can impede successful treatment. In addition, enhancement of cosmetic appearance of the affected nail can be achieved through nail debridement.

It involves the removal of diseased part of the nail using different techniques. These aim at reducing the thickness of the nail, improving its shape, and can aid in the effective penetration of topical antifungal agents into the nail plate. Nail debridement serves as a valuable approach to improve the visual appearance of the affected nail and optimize the efficacy of treatment in addressing onychomycosis [22].

7.4.2 Nail Lacquers and Cosmetics

Cosmetic camouflage has the ability to conceal the cosmetic imperfections resulting from onychomycosis, resulting in an instant enhancement in the appearance of the affected nail. At the same time, one should be watchful of the underlying condition from time to time, as well as careful about potential spread. Nail lacquers with pigments or keratolytic agents can effectively camouflage discoloration and create a smoother nail surface. Nevertheless, it is crucial to recognize that cosmetic measures do not eliminate the underlying infection by themselves. Combining them with antifungal therapy is necessary to achieve optimal outcomes. While cosmetic products provide immediate cosmetic improvement, addressing the fungal infection through appropriate antifungal treatment remains essential for comprehensive management [23].

Toe nail onychomycosis is a prevalent condition among elderly and diabetic patients, who often have underlying health issues, making oral antifungals less suitable. The effectiveness of topical antifungal agents used as standalone treatments is generally limited. However, a novel approach involving regular chemical peeling of nails, in conjunction with topical antifungal nail lacquers, had shown promising results in two cases. Black peel, which contains acetic acid, salicylic acid, jasmonic acid, biosulphur and potassium iodide, exhibits broad-spectrum antimicrobial properties, specifically targeting fungi and biofilms. Combining nail peeling using black peel with the application of topical antifungal medications may lead to enhanced outcomes [24].

7.5 Enhancement of Patient's Quality of Life

Onychomycosis has been shown to have a profound effect on a patient's quality of life, causing feelings of embarrassment, social withdrawal and low self-esteem. Warshaw et al. reported that patients who achieved complete cure of the target toenail experienced a minimum average decrease of 13 points in NailQoL scores compared to those who did not achieve cure. Furthermore, patients who achieved complete cure of all ten toenails demonstrated a minimum average decrease of 16 points in NailQoL scores compared to those without complete cure ($p < 0.01$ and $p < 0.01$). Both these differences were statistically significant and roughly twice the reduction reported by patients who did not attain cure status. The NailQoL component and total scores for patients who achieved mycological cure of the target toenail were not statistically different from those who did not achieve mycological cure of the target toenail. This emphasizes that one of the crucial objectives of treatment is to enhance the patient's overall well-being and psychological state [25].

By addressing the physical symptoms and improving the appearance of the affected nails, treatment aims to alleviate the negative impact on the patient's emotional and social aspects, thus improving the patient's overall quality of life, as a part of comprehensive management of onychomycosis. A recent systematic review of ten randomized controlled trials (RCTs) examining quality-of-life (QoL) outcomes in patients with onychomycosis showed statistically significant improvement from baseline to the end of treatment in all four measures assessing satisfaction with treatment. Mental health also exhibited significant improvement in all three measures. The OnyCOE-t™ and NailQoL are the most commonly used outcome measures to evaluate QoL in these studies [26]. Various components of improvement in overall quality of life of patients with onychomycosis are listed below. These should be important treatment goals.

7.5.1 Symptom Relief

Symptoms such as nail pain, discomfort and malodour can be associated with onychomycosis. A successful treatment approach should focus on alleviating these as well, enhancing the patient's physical comfort and overall quality of life. By effectively addressing the underlying fungal infection, treatment aims to provide relief from the associated discomfort and improve the daily well-being. Improving physical comfort becomes a significant objective in the comprehensive management of onychomycosis, aiming to enhance the overall quality of life for individuals affected by the condition [6].

7.5.2 Patient Counselling and Support

Offering counselling and support to patients can play a valuable role in managing the emotional challenges. By addressing patient concerns, providing clear explanations of treatment expectations and offering reassurance throughout the therapeutic journey, dermatologists can significantly enhance patient satisfaction and promote adherence to therapy. This supportive approach not only helps patients cope with the emotional burden associated but also fosters a stronger therapeutic relationship and encourages active engagement in their own care. By acknowledging and addressing the emotional aspects, dermatologists can promote a positive treatment experience, optimizing patient outcomes [21].

7.5.3 Quality of Life

Several quality-of-life scales have been used to assess the impact of onychomycosis on patients' well-being. These are detailed below.

i. **Nail-Specific Quality-of-Life Questionnaire (NailQoL)**
   This scale is designed to evaluate the impact of nail conditions on patients' quality of life related to nail appearance, self-esteem and psychological well-being. It consists of multiple domains, including symptoms, emotions, social interactions and daily activities. The NailQoL provides a comprehensive assessment of the specific challenges faced by individuals with onychomycosis. The NailQoL questionnaire consists of 15 items categorized into symptom (3), emotion (10) and functional (2) domains (Table 7.5). The symptom and emotion subscales exhibit strong internal consistency, ranging from 0.80 to 0.92. When administered to 46 patients 1 month after baseline, the instrument demonstrated good reproducibility, with an ICC (intraclass correlation coefficient) of 0.88–0.91. In a study involving 292 patients at 18 months, statistically significant improvements in NailQoL scores were observed among individuals who achieved complete cure (both mycological and clinical) ($P<0.01$). The NailQoL questionnaire is a concise, valid, reliable and responsive tool for assessing the impact of onychomycosis on patients' quality of life [25].

ii. **Onychomycosis Quality of Life (OnyQoL)**
   The OnyQoL scale is a disease-specific measure developed to evaluate the impact of onychomycosis on patients' quality of life. It includes domains such as symptoms, functional limitations, emotions and social interactions related to the condition (Table 7.6). The OnyQoL scale captures both physical and psychosocial aspects of onychomycosis, providing valuable insights into patients' experiences [27].

iii. **Dermatology Life Quality Index (DLQI)**
   Although not specific to onychomycosis, the DLQI is a widely used generic scale for assessing quality of life in dermatological conditions. It covers various aspects of patients' lives, including symptoms, daily activities, personal relationships and emotional well-being. The DLQI provides a broad assessment of how skin conditions, including onychomycosis, impact overall quality of life. However, some

TABLE 7.5

NailQoL Questionnaire

Domains	Statements for Scoring[a]
Symptoms	My nail condition hurts.
	The skin around my nails is irritated.
	The skin around my nail and/or nails is sensitive.
Emotion	I worry that my nail condition may be serious.
	I am ashamed of my nail condition.
	I worry that my nail condition may get worse.
	I am embarrassed about my nail condition.
	I am frustrated with my nail condition.
	I am annoyed by my nail condition.
	I have felt frustrated by the lack of improvement of my nails with previous treatment.
	My nails make me feel less attractive.
	My nails make me self-conscious.
	I am worried I may give my nail fungus to other people.
Function	My nails are difficult to cut.
	I rely on other people to help cut my nail.

[a] The scale scores of symptoms, emotion and function are calculated by the average of the item scores that pertain to that particular scale. The items are scored on a 0–100 scale where 0=never; 25=rarely; 50=sometimes; 75=often; 100=all the time.

questions may not be specifically applicable to nail disease including onychomycosis. Also, often the impact of cutaneous fungal infection may be difficult to differentiate from nail fungal infection [28].

iv. **Medical Outcomes Study Short Form 36 (SF-36)**

The SF-36 is a generic health-related quality-of-life scale used across various medical conditions. It assesses several dimensions of health, including physical functioning, social functioning, role limitations and emotional well-being. While not specific to onychomycosis, the SF-36 can provide a broader perspective on patients' overall well-being and the impact of onychomycosis on different aspects of their lives [28].

Each of these scales has its strengths and focuses on different aspects of quality of life in onychomycosis. Disease-specific scales like NailQoL and OnyQoL provide a targeted assessment of the condition's impact, capturing specific concerns related to onychomycosis. Generic scales like DLQI and SF-36 offer a broader evaluation of overall quality of life, allowing comparison with other dermatological and medical conditions. The choice of scale depends on the research or clinical objectives, the need for specificity to onychomycosis, and the desired breadth of assessment. Researchers and healthcare professionals should consider the psychometric properties, applicability and relevance of each scale to ensure accurate and meaningful evaluation of quality of life in onychomycosis patients [25–28].

TABLE 7.6

Onychomycosis Quality-of-Life (OnyQoL) Scale

S. No.	Statements	Scoring Pattern
1	People find it unpleasant to look at my nails. My nails look neglected.	Each item scored on a 5-point scale as follows:
2	I think that other people notice my nail problem.	
3	I feel disheartened because of my nail problem.	• Not at all
4	It costs a lot of money to look after my nails.	• Yes, but this is not bothersome
5	I worry that my nail problem is contagious.	• Yes, this is somewhat bothersome
6	I am upset by the appearance of my nails.	• Yes, this is very bothersome
7	I worry about having this nail problem for the rest of my life.	• Yes, this is extremely bothersome
8	I feel I have to keep my nails cut short.	
9	I can't wear the shoes I want because of my nail problem.	
10	I cannot forget that I have this nail problem.	
11	My nail problem is a nuisance.	
12	I worry this might spread.	
13	My nails are thick and discoloured.	
14	I have difficulty cutting my nails.	
15	I have pain in my toes and nails.	
16	The nail seems to be being eaten away.	
17	My doctor does not show enough concern about my condition.	
18	My doctor is misinformed about how to treat my nail problem.	
19	The treatment I receive is effective.	
20	I worry about the side effects of my treatment.	
21	My treatment is inconvenient.	
22	My treatment is too long.	
23	I am disappointed with my treatment.	
24	I think the treatment is not effective.	
25	I worry about treatment because of the side effects.	
26	I think the treatment is inconvenient.	
27	I think the treatment is too long.	
28	I am disappointed with the treatment.	

Additional Questions	Objective Responses
What is your monthly household income?	
How much of your vacation time would you be willing to sacrifice to get rid of your mycosis once and for all?	
What amount of money would you be willing to spend to get rid of your mycosis once and for all?	

7.6 Preventing Antifungal Resistance

Reports of resistance to antifungal drugs are rising across the globe [29]. It is a multifactorial problem attributable to clinical factors as well as microbiological resistance due to genetic mutations in causative organisms. As of date, resistance to both azoles and terbinafine is well documented. Whenever antifungal resistance is suspected, one should carefully confirm the diagnosis. When confirmed, one should evaluate the probable cause of non-response (drug resistance, noncompliance, structural alterations in the nail). This is important to enable appropriate remedial measures.

Resistance to azoles and terbinafine has been attributed to overexposure to these drugs. Onychomycosis case studies reporting failure to terbinafine are becoming more common [30,31]. Pulse dosing schedules have been considered to be contributory. Prevalence of terbinafine-resistant strains (*Trichophyton rubrum*, *Trichophyton mentagrophytes*, *Trichophyton indotineae*) with SQLE mutations has been reported to account for 16%–77% isolates from dermatophytosis; and this phenomenon is global now [32]. Azole resistance, observed in *Candida* and *Aspergillus* species, is associated with mutations in *ERG11*, *MDR1*, *CDR1* and *CDR2* genes [33]. Global incidence of azole resistance in dermatophytes is roughly 19% [34]. Due to widespread immigration and travel, onychomycosis is also showing a shift towards more of NDMs and mixed infection [30].

NDM and mixed infections should be investigated as possible etiological agents for onychomycosis [21]. This is important especially in cases with treatment failure. Overall, the usage of broad-spectrum antifungals (itraconazole, efinaconazole, tavaborole) may be associated with better treatment response when multiple infections are suspected. Preventive strategies as explained above can also contribute a lot towards prevention of antifungal resistance. Confirming diagnosis of onychomycosis before embarking on prolonged antifungal therapy needs to be emphasized further.

7.7 Conclusions

Treating onychomycosis necessitates a holistic strategy that encompasses the complete elimination of the fungal infection, restoration of nail appearance and function, prevention of relapse and enhancement of patients' psychological and social well-being. By addressing these multiple dimensions of treatment, healthcare professionals can optimize therapeutic outcomes, increase patient satisfaction and enhance the overall management of onychomycosis. It is crucial to foster ongoing research and collaboration to deepen our understanding of this intricate condition and develop more efficacious treatment approaches?.

References

1. Christenson JK, Peterson GM, Naunton M, et al. Challenges and opportunities in the management of onychomycosis. *J Fungi (Basel)*. 2018;4:87.
2. Scher RK, Tavakkol A, Sigurgeirsson B, et al. Onychomycosis: diagnosis and definition of cure. *J Am Acad Dermatol*. 2007;56:939–44.

3. Maskan Bermudez N, Rodríguez-Tamez G, Perez S, et al. Onychomycosis: old and new. *J Fungi (Basel)*. 2023;9:559.
4. Lipner SR, Scher RK. Efinaconazole in the treatment of onychomycosis. *Infect Drug Resist*. 2015 Jun 1;8:163–72.
5. Mahajan K, Grover C, Relhan V, et al. Nail Society of India (NSI) recommendations for pharmacologic therapy of onychomycosis. *Indian Dermatol Online J*. 2023;14:330–41.
6. Leung AKC, Lam JM, Leong KF, et al. Onychomycosis: an updated review. *Recent Pat Inflamm Allergy Drug Discov*. 2020;14:32–45.
7. Falotico JM, Lipner SR. Updated perspectives on the diagnosis and management of onychomycosis. *Clin Cosmet Investig Dermatol*. 2022;15:1933–57.
8. Gupta AK, Stec N. Recent advances in therapies for onychomycosis and its management. *F1000Res*. 2019;8:F1000 Faculty Rev-968.
9. Gupta AK, Lynch LE, Kogan N, et al. The use of an intermittent terbinafine regimen for the treatment of dermatophyte toenail onychomycosis. *J Eur Acad Dermatol Venereol*. 2009;23:256–62.
10. Shemer A, Daniel R, Rigopoulos D, et al. Variability in systemic treatment efficacy for onychomycosis: information that clinical studies do not impart to the office dermatologist. *Skin Appendage Disord*. 2018;4:141–4.
11. Yadav P, Singal A, Pandhi D, et al. Comparative efficacy of continuous and pulse dose terbinafine regimes in toenail dermatophytosis: a randomized double-blind trial. *Indian J Dermatol Venereol Leprol*. 2015 Jul–Aug;81(4):363–9.
12. Carney C, Tosti A, Daniel R, et al. A new classification system for grading the severity of onychomycosis: onychomycosis severity index. *Arch Dermatol*. 2011;147:1277–82.
13. Warshaw EM, Carver SM, Zielke GR, et al. Intermittent terbinafine for toenail onychomycosis: is it effective? Results of a randomized pilot trial. *Arch Dermatol*. 2001;137:1253.
14. Tosti A, Elewski BE. Onychomycosis: practical approaches to minimize relapse and recurrence. *Skin Appendage Disord*. 2016;2:83–7.
15. Scher RK, Baran R. Onychomycosis in clinical practice: factors contributing to recurrence. *Br J Dermatol*. 2003;149:5–9.
16. Elewski BE, Tosti A. Risk factors and comorbidities for onychomycosis: implications for treatment with topical therapy. *J Clin Aesthet Dermatol*. 2015;8:38–42.
17. Gupta AK, Elewski BE, Rosen T, et al. Onychomycosis: strategies to minimize recurrence. *J Drugs Dermatol*. 2016;15:279–82.
18. Gupta AK, Foley KA. Evidence for biofilms in onychomycosis. *G Ital Dermatol Venereol*. 2019;154:50–5.
19. Shemer A, Gupta AK, Kamshov A, et al. Topical antifungal treatment prevents recurrence of toenail onychomycosis following cure. *Dermatol Ther*. 2017;30:e12545.
20. Vlahovic TC, Gupta AK. Efinaconazole topical solution (10%) for the treatment of onychomycosis in adult and pediatric patients. *Expert Rev Anti Infect Ther*. 2022;20:3–15.
21. Gupta AK, Venkataraman M, Renaud HJ, et al. A paradigm shift in the treatment and management of onychomycosis. *Skin Appendage Disord*. 2021;7:351–8.
22. Malay DS, Yi S, Borowsky P, et al. Efficacy of debridement alone versus debridement combined with topical antifungal nail lacquer for the treatment of pedal onychomycosis: a randomized, controlled trial. *J Foot Ankle Surg*. 2009;48:294–308.
23. Akhtar N, Sharma H, Pathak K. Onychomycosis: potential of nail lacquers in transungual delivery of antifungals. *Scientifica (Cairo)*. 2016;2016:1387936.
24. Sonthalia S, Jakhar D, Yadav P, et al. Chemical peeling as an innovative treatment alternative to oral antifungals for onychomycosis in special circumstances. *Skin Appendage Disord*. 2019;5:181–5.
25. Warshaw EM, Foster JK, Cham PM, et al. NailQoL: a quality-of-life instrument for onychomycosis. *Int J Dermatol*. 2007;46:1279–86.
26. Wang J, Wiznia LE, Rieder EA. Patient-reported outcomes in onychomycosis: a review of psychometrically evaluated instruments in assessing treatment effectiveness. *Skin Appendage Disord*. 2017;3:144–5.

27. Milobratović D, Janković S, Vukičević J, et al. Quality of life in patients with toenail onychomycosis. *Mycoses*. 2013;56:543–51.

28. Szepietowski JC, Reich A. National quality of life in dermatology group. Stigmatisation in onychomycosis patients: a population-based study. *Mycoses*. 2009;52:343–9.

29. Gupta AK, Renaud HJ, Quinlan EM, et al. The growing problem of antifungal resistance in onychomycosis and other superficial mycoses. *Am J Clinic Dermatol*. 2021;22:149–57.

30. Nofal A, Fawzy MM, El-Hawary EE. Successful treatment of resistant onychomycosis with voriconazole in a liver transplant patient. *Dermatol Ther*. 2020;33:e14014.

31. Kimura U, Hiruma M, Kano R, et al. Onychomycosis caused by *Scopulariopsis brevicaulis*: the third documented case in Japan. *J Dermatol*. 2019;46:e167–8.

32. Ebert A, Monod M, Salamin K, et al. Alarming India-wide phenomenon of antifungal resistance in dermatophytes: a multicentre study. *Mycoses*. 2020;63:717–28.

33. Ksiezopolska E, Gabaldón T. Evolutionary emergence of drug resistance in *Candida* opportunistic pathogens. *Genes*. 2018;9:461.

34. Ghannoum M. Azole resistance in dermatophytes: prevalence and mechanism of action. *J Am Podiat Med Assoc*. 2016;106:79–86.

8

Current Treatments of Onychomycosis

Michelle S. Bach and Elizabeth Yim

8.1 Introduction

Onychomycosis is difficult to treat due to the location of infection in the nail plate, low patient adherence due to long treatment duration and lower efficacy rates of existing therapies [1]. Recurrence rates can range from 6.5% to 53%, and some patients may exhibit permanent nail changes even after treatment [2]. Despite these challenges in treatment, a variety of topical, oral and physical therapies are available, with novel therapies currently in the pipeline [3]. Therefore, this chapter will highlight existing treatment options available for onychomycosis.

Goals of treatment include mycological cure defined as negative fungal culture or potassium hydroxide (KOH) test or Periodic acid–Schiff (PAS) stain as well as complete cure defined as no nail involvement on examination and a negative fungal culture, KOH or PAS stain [4,5]. There are several topical and oral therapies for onychomycosis approved in the United States (US) and Europe as well as off-label and mechanical treatment options (Table 8.1). These types of treatment will be described in more detail throughout this chapter. The appropriate treatment for the patient will depend on patient characteristics, comorbidities, clinical severity and interactions with medications (Table 8.2).

8.2 Treatments: Topical Therapies

Topical medication can be used for the treatment of onychomycosis, such as dermatophytomas, superficial onychomycosis, and for distal lateral subungual onychomycosis (DSLO) involving one or few digits with less than 50% of the nail surface without matrix involvement . Topical treatment is also an option for paediatric patients whose nails grow rapidly as well as for patients where oral antifungals are contraindicated. They are also used for maintenance therapy and preventing recurrence. The main advantage of topical treatment is that there is no risk of systemic side effects as well as no drug interactions. The most common adverse effects are skin irritation, pruritus, burning sensation, and periungual erythema, usually at the site of application [6].

DOI: 10.1201/9781003381648-9

TABLE 8.1

Oral and Topical Treatments for Onychomycosis

Orals	Topicals
Terbinafine	Ciclopirox 8% lacquer
Itraconazole	Tavaborole 5% solution
Griseofulvin[a]	Efinaconazole 10% solution
Fluconazole[b]	Amorolfine 5% lacquer[c]
	Luliconazole 5% solution[d]

[a] No longer recommended for the treatment of onychomycosis in adults.
[b] Oral fluconazole is used off-label in the US while it is approved in Europe for onychomycosis.
[c] Approved in Europe only.
[d] Luliconazole 5% solution is approved for topical treatment of onychomycosis in Japan.

TABLE 8.2

Determining Factors for Onychomycosis Treatment

Patient Characteristics	Comorbidities	Nail Presentation	Medications
Paediatric Patients (Check Other Family Members)	Peripheral vascular disease	Mild: <20% involvement	Benzodiazepines
Advancing Age	Immunosuppression	Moderate: 20%–60%	Hydrochlorothiazide
Pregnancy	Uncontrolled diabetes	Severe: >60%	Statins
Breastfeeding	Hepatic disease	Dermatophytoma	Warfarin
	Renal disease	Mixed infections	Others

8.3 Ciclopirox

Ciclopirox 8% nail lacquer was the first topical treatment to be approved by the FDA for the treatment of mild to moderate onychomycosis for those who are at least 12 years of age or older [7]. Ciclopirox is hypothesized to inhibit degradation of peroxides in the fungal cell by chelating polyvalent cations and has antifungal activity against dermatophytes, non-dermatophytic fungi and *Candida* species [8,9]. The recommended frequency of application is once daily to the nail plate and surrounding skin for 24 weeks (fingernail onychomycosis) or 48 weeks (toenail onychomycosis) [10,11]. As a lacquer, the drug reaches the site of infection via the transungual route, penetrating the nail plate to reach the nail bed and inhibiting germination of spores. Patients should be instructed to trim and file the nails weekly during treatment [12]. The mycologic cure rate of 29%–36% and complete cure rate of 5.5%–8.5% are lower than those observed with systemic treatment as well as with newer topicals such as efinaconazole (Table 8.3) [8]. Despite the low cure rates and long treatment duration, the advantages of avoiding hepatotoxicity and the low levels of resistance make ciclopirox an appealing therapeutic option [7,10,13].

8.4 Amorolfine

Amorolfine 5% nail lacquer is a morpholine that inhibits delta-14 reductase and delta-7–delta-8 isomerase involved in ergosterol synthesis [14]. Amorolfine is not FDA approved

TABLE 8.3

Complete and Mycologic Cure Rates for Onychomycosis Topical Therapies [8,16,18,19,23,32,34,36]

Topical Therapy	Pregnancy Category	Treatment Duration	Mycologic Cure Rate	Complete Cure Rate
Ciclopirox 8% lacquer[a]	B	Once daily for 48 weeks	29%–36%	5.5%–8.5%
Tavaborole 5% solution[a]	C	Once daily for 48 weeks	31.1%–35.9%	6.5%–9.1%
Efinaconazole 10% solution[a]	C	Once daily for 48 weeks	53.4%–55.2%	15.2%–17.8%
Amorolfine 5% lacquer[b]	Not reported	Twice weekly for 24 weeks	71.2%–75.3%	45.6%–51.8%
Luliconazole 5% solution[a]	Not reported	Once daily for 48 weeks	45.4%	14.9%

[a] Complete cure defined as 0% clinical involvement of the target nail, negative KOH and negative culture.
[b] Complete cure rates for amorolfine were defined as <10% nail involvement and not by the standard definition of zero nail involvement on examination.

in the US but is approved in Europe for the treatment of onychomycosis [15,16]. The recommended frequency of application is once or twice weekly for 6 months (fingernail onychomycosis) or 9–12 months (toenail onychomycosis) [15]. Based on prior randomized controlled trials (RCTs), complete cure rates ranged from 45.6% to 51.8% and mycological cure rates ranged from 71.2% to 75.3% (Table 8.3) [12,17–19]. Complete cure rate for amorolfine was defined as <10% nail involvement and not by the standard definition of zero nail involvement on examination [20]. The most common adverse effects are nail damage, nail discoloration, dryness, burning sensation, pruritus and erythema [6,21]. According to a study on the cost-effectiveness of topical antifungal therapies for onychomycosis, amorolfine was considered more cost-effective (cost per patient: 84 Euros) than ciclopirox (cost per patient: 252 Euros) [22].

8.5 Tavaborole

Tavaborole 5% solution is a new benzoxazole that inhibits aminoacyl-transfer ribonucleic acid synthetase involved in fungal protein synthesis [23]. Tavaborole is FDA approved for the treatment of dermatophytic toenail onychomycosis in patients ≥6 years of age. It is most effective against *Trichophyton rubrum* and *Trichophyton mentagrophytes* [24]. The recommended frequency of application on the toenail is once daily for 48 weeks [23]. The most common adverse effects are dermatitis, ingrown toenail, exfoliation and erythema [12,24–26]. FDA-reported complete cure rates ranged from 6.5% to 9.1% while mycological cure rates ranged from 31.1% to 35.9%, similar to those of ciclopirox (Table 8.3) [23]. Due to its smaller molecular weight, tavaborole exhibits higher penetration through the nail plate compared to ciclopirox or amorolfine [27–29]. The main limitation of tavaborole is high cost and limited insurance coverage. The cost of a 10 mL bottle of tavaborole is ~$1500.00 [30].

8.6 Efinaconazole

Efinaconazole 10% solution is a new azole that inhibits lanosterol 14α-demethylase necessary for ergosterol synthesis [20,31]. Efinaconazole is FDA approved for the treatment of toenail onychomycosis in patients ≥18 years of age [32]. The recommended frequency of application is the same as tavaborole – once daily for 48 weeks [32]. It has been found to be particularly successful in treating dermatophytomas [33]. Efinaconazole should be applied to the nail plate, nail folds, hyponychium and underside of the nail plate [13,32,34]. The most common adverse effects reported are dermatitis, pain, onychocryptosis and vesiculation [20]. Efinaconazole exhibits superior penetration of the nail plate and currently has the highest reported cure rates out of all topicals approved for onychomycosis, with FDA-reported mycological cure rate around 53.4%–55.2% and complete cure rate around 15.2%–17.8% (Table 8.3). Its main limitations are high cost and lack of insurance coverage – a 4 mL bottle of efinaconazole is estimated to cost ~$600.

8.7 Luliconazole 5% Solution

Topical luliconazole is approved for use in Japan but not in the US for onychomycosis. It is an imidazole antifungal with fungicidal activity against both dermatophytes and non-dermatophytes, with higher potency than amorolfine, ciclopirox and terbinafine based on in vitro studies [35]. A multicentre, phase III RCT conducted in Japan reported a complete cure rate of 14.9% and mycologic cure rate of 45.4% after once-daily treatment for 48 weeks (Table 8.3) [36,37].

8.8 Topical Treatment for Paediatric Patients

Onychomycosis is less commonly seen in children than in adults, and close attention should be paid to additional family members for onychomycosis if a child presents with onychomycosis (Figure 8.1). At present, ciclopirox 8% lacquer is FDA approved for the treatment of onychomycosis in patients ≥12 years of age. Tavaborole 5% topical solution and efinaconazole 10% topical solution are FDA approved for the treatment of onychomycosis in patients ≥6 years of age [38,39]. Paediatric patients may respond better to topical treatment than adults due to a faster nail growth, smaller nail surface area and lower prevalence of tinea pedis (Table 8.4) [8,23,32,38,40–44]. While guidelines for topical treatment in paediatrics are the same as for adults, clinical and complete cures may be achieved sooner in children.

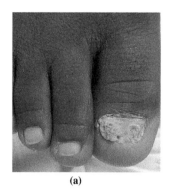 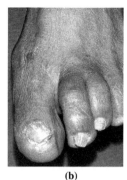

| (a)   (b) |

FIGURE 8.1

(a) 11-year-old male with confirmed onychomycosis (positive fungal culture and positive KOH) with total involvement of entire nail plate, including nail matrix. In a paediatric patient presenting with onychomycosis, close examination of family members is important. (b) Examination of mother's digits revealed that mother also had long-standing onychomycosis (positive fungal culture and KOH) and tinea pedis for several years. Both child and mother were initiated on oral antifungals.

TABLE 8.4

FDA-Approved Topical Agents, Dosing Regimen and Cure Rates for Paediatric Onychomycosis [8,23,32,38,40–43,114,138]

Topical Therapy	Study	Age	Dosing	Mycologic Cure Rate	Complete Cure Rate
Ciclopirox 8% lacquer[a]	Prospective, randomized, double-blind	2–16	Once daily for 32 weeks	77%	34.2%
Tavaborole 5% solution[b]	Phase IV, single arm, open-label	6–16	Once daily for 48 weeks	36.2%	8.5%
Efinaconazole 10% solution[c]	Phase IV, multicentre, open-label (40)	6–16	Once daily for 48 weeks	65%	40%

[a] Clinical cure defined as negative culture and Investigator Global Assessment (IGA) score of 0 (42).
[b] Clinical cure defined as ≤ 5% dystrophic or discoloured distal toenail plate with minimal onycholysis and subungual hyperkeratosis (41).
[c] Clinical cure defined as zero clinical involvement and mycological cure (40).

8.9 Alternative Topicals

There are few studies investigating the use of alternative topicals to treat onychomycosis, such as thymol, tea tree oil, Vicks VapoRub™ (The Proctor & Gamble Company, Cincinnati, OH), arthrospira maxima, ozonized sunflower oil, natural coniferous resin lacquer and vitamin E [45]. Many of these clinical studies are limited either due to a small sample size or have lower efficacy rates than current approved treatments. While larger clinical trials are needed, these alternative treatments are often associated with low risks and may even be used in combination with systemic treatment to increase efficacy and reduce recurrence [45–53].

8.10 Treatments: Oral Therapies

While topicals can be considered for mild to moderate onychomycosis, most topicals have a lower cure rate than systemic treatments due to poor penetration of the drug in the nail plate and decreased access to the nail bed, especially when there is hyperkeratosis. In addition, the long treatment duration with topicals makes patient adherence more challenging. When there is more severe nail involvement such as >50% of the nail plate, nail matrix involvement, multiple digits involved, total nail dystrophy, systemic treatment should be considered.

8.11 Terbinafine

Terbinafine is the first-line treatment for onychomycosis due to its higher mycological cure rate of 70% compared to itraconazole's 44% observed in clinical trials (Table 8.5) [54,55]. Terbinafine, an inhibitor of squalene epoxidase, is fungistatic by preventing the formation of ergosterol in the cell membrane and fungicidal due to the toxic accumulation of squalene [56,57]. Terbinafine is most effective against dermatophytic onychomycosis compared to yeasts and non-dermatophytic infections [58].

The recommended dosage and duration of treatment is one 250 mg tablet once daily for 6 weeks for onychomycosis of the fingernails and 12 weeks for onychomycosis of the toenails [59]. Alternative treatment schedules include taking one 250 mg tablet twice daily for 1 week every 3 months or two pulse cycles of 250 mg daily for 4 weeks followed by 4 weeks off [60–62]. Pulse dosing may be considered to be safer in patients with comorbidities, and may even be more cost-effective [27].

TABLE 8.5

Complete and Mycologic Cure Rates for Onychomycosis Oral Therapies (72,87,88,93)

Oral Therapy	Pregnancy Category	Treatment Duration	Mycologic Cure Rate	Complete Cure Rate
Terbinafine	B	Fingernail: 250 mg, one tablet, once daily for 6 weeks Toenail: 250 mg, one tablet, once daily for 12 weeks	Fingernail: 79% Toenail: 70%	Fingernail: 59% Toenail: 38%
Itraconazole	C	Fingernail: 200 mg, one tablet, twice per day for 1 week (pulse), followed by 3 weeks without itraconazole, followed by a second week (pulse) of 200 mg, one tablet, twice per day Toenail: 200 mg, one tablet, once daily for 12 weeks	Fingernail: 61% Toenail: 54%	Fingernail: 47% Toenail: 14%
Fluconazole	D	100–450 mg once weekly for 12 to 48 weeks	47%, 59% and 62% at 4, 6 or 9 months of treatment	28%, 29% and 36% at 4, 6 or 9 months of treatment

Adverse effects include elevated transaminases and hepatotoxicity as well as lympho-cytopenia, the latter of which can be seen more in immunosuppressed patients [54,59,63]. Terbinafine is metabolized by the liver and inhibits CYP2D6; therefore, it is important that physicians perform a thorough medication review of their patients for any drug interactions. Terbinafine may increase drug levels of tricyclic antidepressants, selective serotonin reuptake inhibitors (SSRIs), monoamine oxidase inhibitors (MAOIs), and beta-blockers (Table 8.6) [64,65]. Other drug interactions include increasing levels of warfarin and cyclosporine and decreasing levels of terbinafine when taken with rifampin, phenobarbital and cimetidine [54,66]. The most common adverse effects are headaches followed by gastrointestinal disturbances including diarrhoea and dyspepsia, then dermatological symptoms including rash and pruritus, and liver enzyme irregularities [59].

TABLE 8.6

FDA-Reported Drug-Drug Interactions for Oral Therapies for Onychomycosis [72,93,94]

Oral Therapy	Drug Interaction	Effect
Terbinafine	Tricyclic antidepressants	Terbinafine is a CYP450 2D6 inhibitor. Drugs listed on the left are metabolized by CYP450 2D6.
	Selective serotonin reuptake inhibitors	
	Beta-blockers	
	Antiarrhythmics Class 1C (flecainide, propafenone)	
	Monoamine oxidase inhibitors type B	
	Cyclosporine	Increases cyclosporine clearance by 15%.
	Fluconazole	Increases levels of terbinafine.
	Rifampin	Increases terbinafine clearance by 100%. Rifampin is a CYP450 inducer.
	Cimetidine	Decreases terbinafine clearance by 33%. Cimetidine is a CYP450 inhibitor.
Itraconazole	Methadone	Itraconazole increases plasma levels of the drugs listed on the left.
	Disopyramide	
	Dofetilide	
	Dronedarone	
	Quinidine	
	Isavuconazole	
	Ergot alkaloids (e.g. dihydroergotamine, ergometrine [ergonovine], ergotamine, methylergometrine [methylergonovine])	
	Irinotecan	
	Lurasidone	
	Oral midazolam	
	Pimozide	
	Triazolam	
	Felodipine	
	Nisoldipine	

(Continued)

TABLE 8.6 (*Continued*)

FDA-Reported Drug-Drug Interactions for Oral Therapies for Onychomycosis [72,93,94]

Oral Therapy	Drug Interaction	Effect
	Ivabradine	
	Ranolazine	
	Eplerenone	
	Cisapride	
	Naloxegol	
	Lomitapide	
	Lovastatin	
	Simvastatin	
	Avanafil	
	Ticagrelor	
	Colchicine	Contraindicated in patients with renal or hepatic impairments.
	Fesoterodine	
	Solifenacin	
	Eliglustat	Contraindicated in patients on strong or moderate CYP2D6 inhibitors.
Fluconazole	Levonorgestrel	Fluconazole may lead to slight increases in levonorgestrel and ethinyl estradiol.
	Ethinyl estradiol	
	Cimetidine	May lead to a decrease in fluconazole levels.
	Hydrochlorothiazide	May lead to an increase in fluconazole levels.
	Rifampin	May lead to a decrease in fluconazole levels and an increase in fluconazole clearance.
	Warfarin	May lead to a significant increase in prothrombin time.
	Phenytoin	May lead to an increase in the plasma levels of the drug listed on the left.
	Cyclosporine	
	Zidovudine	
	Theophylline	
	Terfenadine	
	Quinidine	
	Oral hypoglycaemics	
	Tolbutamide	
	Glipizide	
	Glyburide	
	Rifabutin	
	Tacrolimus	
	Cisapride	
	Midazolam	
	Voriconazole	
	Tofacitinib	

In an open-label, multicentre trial, the average mycological cure rate at 6 months was 77% and complete cure rate was 44.6% [67]. According to a meta-analysis of RCTs, the mycological cure rate was 76% and complete cure rate was 66% [68]. Terbinafine exhibits higher mycological and complete cure rates and lower recurrence rates compared to itraconazole and higher mycological cure rate than fluconazole [69,70].

8.12 Itraconazole

Itraconazole, an inhibitor of cytochrome P450-dependent 14-α demethylase necessary for ergosterol synthesis, is fungistatic against *Candida* species, dermatophytes and non-dermatophytic fungi [58,71]. Itraconazole is FDA approved for the treatment of *T. rubrum* and *T. mentagrophytes* toenail onychomycosis and dermatophyte-associated fingernail onychomycosis [72,73]. While itraconazole has lower efficacy than terbinafine in treating dermatophytic onychomycosis, in vitro studies have shown that itraconazole has better efficacy than terbinafine for non-dermatophyte moulds.

The recommended dosage and duration of treatment for toenail onychomycosis is one 200 mg tablet once daily with a full meal (high gastric pH for better absorption) at the same time of day for 12 continuous weeks [72]. Alternative treatment schedules include pulse dosing of 3–4 cycles of 200 mg twice daily for a total of 400 mg per day for 1 week per month [74]. For fingernail onychomycosis, treatment is two cycles of 200 mg twice daily for 1 week per month [58,73]. Patients with decreased gastric acidity due to antacids or achlorhydria may exhibit lower rates of itraconazole absorption [75,76].

Itraconazole is contraindicated in patients with ventricular dysfunction, including congestive heart failure, or a history of congestive heart failure [73,77]. All patients should be monitored for signs and symptoms of heart failure [78]. Laboratory monitoring for itraconazole includes serum transaminases prior to initiation in patients with a history of hepatic abnormalities or drug-associated hepatotoxicity and considered for all other patients [73,79]. Consistent blood glucose monitoring is recommended for patients taking concurrent oral hypoglycaemics [80]. Itraconazole has not been adequately investigated in patients with renal insufficiencies [81]. Itraconazole is a potent CYP3A4 inhibitor; therefore, HMG-CoA reductase inhibitors including lovastatin and simvastatin, ergot alkaloids including dihydroergotamine, ergometrine, ergotamine and methylergometrine as well as quinidine, oral midazolam, felodipine, dofetilide, triazolam, pimozide, cisapride, methadone and levacetylmethadol are all contraindicated (Table 8.6) [4,58,73,82]. The most common adverse effects of gastrointestinal disturbances include nausea, vomiting, and diarrhoea, fever, malaise, rash, pruritus, headache, dizziness, hypertension, hypokalaemia, decreased libido and liver enzyme irregularities [73,83].

FDA-reported mycological cure rate for toenail onychomycosis was 54%, complete cure rate was 14% and relapse rate was 21% (Table 8.5). For fingernail onychomycosis, the mycological cure rate was 61% and complete cure rate was 47% [68,73]. According to a meta-analysis of six randomized controlled trials (RCTs), the mycological cure rate of itraconazole was 63%, which was lower than that of terbinafine at 76% but higher than that of fluconazole at 48% [68].

8.13 Fluconazole

Fluconazole, an inhibitor of lanosterol 14α-demethylase necessary for ergosterol synthesis, is currently FDA approved for the treatment of vaginal candidiasis, oropharyngeal and oesophageal candidiasis, and cryptococcal meningitis [84,85]. Although fluconazole is not FDA approved for the treatment of onychomycosis, it is commonly used off-label to treat toenail and fingernail onychomycosis due to its fungistatic activity against dermatophytes and *Candida* species [86]. It is approved in Europe for the treatment of onychomycosis.

The dosage and duration of treatment based on prior RCTs range from 100 to 450 mg weekly for 12–48 weeks with higher mycological and clinical cure rates seen when treatment duration was at least 6 months compared to trials in which duration was less than 6 months [87]. Because fluconazole is renally cleared, patients with impaired renal function will require adjusted dosing based on creatinine levels [82].

There are no established guidelines regarding laboratory monitoring of serum transaminases for fluconazole treatment of onychomycosis [12,16]. Fluconazole has a safer side-effect profile compared to terbinafine and itraconazole and has a long half-life, and can be given weekly dosing. It is a potent inhibitor of CYP2C9 and CYP2C19 and a moderate inhibitor of CYP3A4; therefore, patients who take medications that are metabolized by these enzymes, including but not limited to warfarin, statins, rifampin, phenytoin, zidovudine and calcium channel antagonists, should be closely monitored (Table 8.6) [82,84]. The most common adverse effects were gastrointestinal disturbances including diarrhoea, headache, rash and liver enzyme irregularities [88,89].

In a multicentre RCT, onychomycosis patients received fluconazole 450 mg once weekly for 4, 6 or 9 months with mycologic cure rates of 47%, 59% and 62% and complete cure rates of 28%, 29% and 36%, respectively (Table 8.5) [88]. Additional RCTs have demonstrated mycologic cure rates ranging from 36% to 100%; however, in comparative studies of fluconazole, terbinafine and itraconazole, fluconazole exhibited the lowest mycological cure rates [70,90–92].

8.14 Pregnancy and Breastfeeding

There are no current recommendations for pregnant and breastfeeding patients with onychomycosis; therefore, delaying treatment until afterwards may be safer. Ciclopirox and terbinafine are pregnancy category B; tavaborole, efinaconazole and itraconazole are category C; and fluconazole is category D (Tables 8.3 and 8.5) [8,23,32,72,93,94].

8.15 Systemic Treatment for Paediatrics

Topical treatment can be used as monotherapy in paediatric patients when a single nail is involved, <50% nail plate is involved or there is no matrix involved. However, when multiple nails are involved, >50% nail plate is involved, or there is matrix involvement, oral treatment may be warranted. Griseofulvin, a fungistatic inhibitor of microtubule assembly to prevent fungal replication, was the first FDA-approved oral antifungal therapy for onychomycosis; however, it is no longer prescribed for onychomycosis in adults due to long duration of treatment, adverse effects and high relapse rates [95–97]. Although griseofulvin is no longer recommended in adults, it is FDA approved for paediatric patients with onychomycosis who are ≥2 years of age [98].

Other systemic treatments such as terbinafine and itraconazole can be used off-label and weight-based if warranted, and patient has failed topical treatment and griseofulvin (Table 8.7) [38,99–101].

TABLE 8.7

Recommended Oral Therapies and Dosing Regimen for Paediatric Onychomycosis [38,39,59,69,82,99,100,139–144]

Oral Therapy	Weight	Dosing	Treatment Duration
Griseofulvin	≥2 years old		
	16–27 kg	125–187.5 mg daily	Until nail grows out: ~9–18 months
	>27 kg	187.5–375 mg daily	
Terbinafine	Terbinafine 250 mg tablets		
	<20 kg	62.5 mg/day (1/4 tablet)	Fingernails: 6 weeks Toenails: 12 weeks
	20–40 kg	125 mg/day (1/2 tablet)	
	>40 kg	250 mg/day (1/2 tablet)	
	Terbinafine granules 125 mg or 187.5 mg packet		
	<25 kg	125 mg/day (1 packet of 125 mg)	Fingernails: 6 weeks Toenails: 12 weeks
	25–35 kg	187.5 mg/day (1 packet of 187.5 mg)	
	>35 kg	250 mg/day (2 packets of 125 mg)	
Itraconazole	Continuous therapy		
	100 mg capsule (5 mg/kg/day)		
	10–20 kg	50 mg/day (1/2 of 100 mg capsule on alternate days)	Fingernails: 6 weeks Toenails: 12 weeks
	20–30 kg	100 mg/day (1 capsule of 100 mg each day)	
	30–40 kg	150 mg/day (1 capsule alternating with 2 capsules of size 100 mg)	
	>40 kg	200 mg/day (2 capsules of 100 mg per day)	
	Pulse therapy		
	100 mg capsule (5 mg/kg/day)		
	10–20 kg	50 mg/day (1/2 of 100 mg capsule on alternate days) × 1-week pulse	Fingernail: 2 pulses Toenails: 3 pulses
	20–30 kg	100 mg/day (1 capsule of 100 mg each day) × 1-week pulse	
	30–40 kg	150 mg/day (1 capsule alternating with 2 capsules of size 100 mg) × 1-week pulse	
	40–49 kg	200 mg/day (2 capsules of 100 mg per day) × 1-week pulse	
	>50 kg	400 mg/day (4 capsules of 100 mg per day) × 1-week pulse	
Fluconazole	Intermittent once-weekly therapy		Once weekly until affected nail plate grows out. Fingernails: 12–16 weeks Toenails: 18–26 weeks
	Tablets of 50 mg, 100 mg, 150 mg, 200 mg (6 mg/kg/week)		

8.16 Laboratory Monitoring

Baseline transaminase levels should be obtained prior to starting treatment with oral antifungals. Complete blood count in immunosuppressed patients prescribed terbinafine may be necessary due to the risk of temporary lymphocytopenia [54,59,63]. There has been much debate regarding lab monitoring during treatment with these medications, with several studies finding that lab abnormalities in healthy adults are few and rare during treatment [59,60]. According to a study of 4985 patients taking terbinafine or griseofulvin for dermatophyte infections, there were very infrequent laboratory abnormalities of elevated transaminases, anaemia, lymphopenia and neutropenia, and the few cases (<1% of cases) with abnormalities were of low grade. In a retrospective study of 944 onychomycosis patients on oral terbinafine, 2.4% of patients had abnormal baseline liver function tests, 2.4% of patients had abnormal monitoring liver function tests and no patient had grade 3 or 4 changes indicative of more severe hepatic abnormality [102]. Laboratory abnormalities in patients without prior hepatic damage resolved before treatment completion. Patients who were found to have lab abnormalities were also older (three times more likely to be 65 years or older). Therefore, routine laboratory testing may be unnecessary in patients taking oral antifungal therapies for onychomycosis, especially if they are young (<65 years old) with no pre-existing conditions [103]. It is recommended that in addition to obtaining baseline labs, physicians should screen every patient for liver and haematologic conditions to determine if monitoring is warranted. In high-litigation environments in countries like the US, all patients should be counselled and informed about the potential adverse effects of antifungal therapy, and lab monitoring is based on the discretion of the provider and their patients' comorbidities and medications. If serum transaminases are ordered, ordering alanine transaminase (ALT) only and not a comprehensive liver function test may be more cost-effective as ALT has a longer half-life [104,105].

8.17 Booster Therapy

Booster therapy, defined as 4 weeks of additional oral antifungal medication at 6–9 months after initiation of therapy, has been shown to improve cure rates in patients who do not respond well to the initial course [106]. Patients with immunosuppression, peripheral arterial disease where there is decreased concentration of drug reaching the nails, slow growing nails, thicker nails (>2 mm), lateral involvement, matrix involvement and/or large surface area of infected nail are more likely to benefit from booster therapy [11,107,108].

8.18 Prevention

With recurrence rates of up to 53% reported in the literature, prevention of onychomycosis is key. Recurrence is highest within the first 3 years after completing treatment [96]. High-risk individuals include athletes, diabetics and patients with peripheral arterial disease. Preventative measures include discarding and disinfecting prior footwear, cleaning and drying hands and feet, avoiding walking bare feet in public locations, selecting licensed nail salons and not sharing nail clippers [2,109]. Prophylactic treatment with topicals can also reduce recurrence. Patient awareness and education is key for a prompt diagnosis and for treatment of family members who have tinea pedis or onychomycosis [109].

8.19 Alternative Oral Therapies

The following oral medications are not FDA approved for onychomycosis, but studies have shown mycologic cure rates similar to terbinafine, but higher clinical cure rates compared to terbinafine can be used as alternative treatments should patients fail treatment with standard antifungals (Table 8.8). They are not, however, without side effects, and have several drug interactions one should be aware of, and may require lab monitoring. Although not commonly used as treatment for onychomycosis, with increasing incidence of antifungal resistance, these medications can be used as alternative or adjunct therapy for onychomycosis.

Posaconazole, a triazole similar to itraconazole, was FDA approved in 2006 as prophylaxis for invasive *Aspergillus* and *Candida* in immunocompromised patients [110,111]. Posaconazole is an inhibitor of lanosterol 14α-demethylase, an enzyme involved in the synthesis of ergosterol [112]. As a CYP3A4 inhibitor, posaconazole should not be taken with midazolam or other drugs that involve the CYP3A4 pathway [113]. A phase IIB RCT showed posaconazole 200 mg once daily for 24 weeks to be safe and effective, exhibiting higher complete cure rates than terbinafine (Table 8.8) [114]. A few patients stopped the study based on the protocol due to elevated liver enzymes [114].

Fosravuconazole, a triazole prodrug of ravuconazole, is approved for onychomycosis treatment in Japan but not in the US [115]. In a single institution, retrospective study, 36 patients who did not respond to topical therapies took 100 mg once daily for an average of 11 weeks with ~60% improvement 48 weeks after initiating treatment [116]. The most common adverse effect was elevated transaminases followed by gastrointestinal disturbances. A multicentre RCT of 101 patients who took 100 mg once daily for 12 weeks demonstrated mycological cure rate of 82% and complete cure rate of 59.4% at 48 weeks since initiating treatment (Table 8.8) [117].

TABLE 8.8

Alternative Oral Therapies for Onychomycosis [39,114,116–118,121–123,145,146]

Oral Therapy	Dose and Treatment Duration	Mycologic Cure Rate	Complete Cure Rate
Posaconazole	200 mg/day × 24 weeks	70.3%	54.1%
Fosravuconazole	100 mg/day × 12 weeks	82%	59.4%
Voriconazole	400 mg twice a day (loading dose), then 200 mg twice a day for 12 weeks	Not reported	Not reported
Albaconazole	400 mg/week for 36 weeks	34%–71%	16%–34%
Oteseconazole (VT-1161)	300 mg/day × 2 weeks followed by 300 mg/week × 10 weeks	61%–72%	32%–42%

Voriconazole, an inhibitor of lanosterol 14α-demethylation necessary for ergosterol synthesis, is currently FDA approved in patients at least 2 years of age for the treatment of invasive aspergillosis, oesophageal candidiasis, candidemia and other severe fungal infections [118]. Most common adverse effects include visual disturbances, fever, gastrointestinal symptoms, abnormal transaminase levels and tachycardia [118]. A case report of a liver transplant patient with treatment-resistant onychomycosis treated with 200 mg of voriconazole twice daily for 3 months describes complete cure 3 months after initiating treatment (Table 8.8) [119]. There are no RCTs on the safety and efficacy of voriconazole for onychomycosis.

Albaconazole, a novel broad-spectrum triazole, is not currently FDA approved; however, a recent phase II RCT was completed on the safety and efficacy of albaconazole 100–400 mg weekly for 24 or 36 weeks for the treatment of distal subungual onychomycosis (Table 8.8) [120,121]. Dose-dependent clinical cure rates ranged from 16% to 34% and mycological cure rates ranged from 34% to 71%. The most common adverse effects were headaches, gastrointestinal disturbances including diarrhoea, upper respiratory infections, elevated transaminases in 2% of patients and elevated creatine phosphokinase in 2% of patients [121].

Oteseconazole, an inhibitor of 14α-demethylase necessary for ergosterol synthesis, is currently FDA approved for the treatment of vulvovaginal candidiasis [122,123]. Oteseconazole should not be taken concomitantly with breast cancer resistance protein substrates due to elevated levels of the substrates [122]. In a multicentre phase II RCT, patients with DLSO were treated with either oteseconazole 300 mg or 600 mg once daily for 2 weeks then once weekly for 10 or 22 weeks [39,124]. The dose-dependent complete cure rate ranged from 32% to 42%. Mycological cure rates ranged from 61% to 72% at 48 weeks (Table 8.8) [124]. The most common adverse effects were nausea and constipation with no evidence of elevated transaminases or cardiac arrythmias [124].

8.20 Mechanical Therapies

Laser therapies, hypothesized to cause photothermal destruction of fungi, are currently FDA approved for the "temporary increase of clear nail", defined as visual or aesthetic improvement in presentation, but not for a cure of onychomycosis (Figure 8.2) [125]. Prior studies have demonstrated an average mycological cure rate of 11% (in studies following single nail) and 63% (in studies following multiple nails), and an average complete cure rate of 13% [126]. However, several of the studies were not blinded, randomized nor controlled; therefore, there is insufficient evidence to recommend lasers as therapeutic versus cosmetic treatment [127,128]. Lasers used for treatment include 1064 nm Nd:YAG, fractional CO_2, dual diode, and 870 nm, 930 nm and 1320 nm wavelength lasers [126,129]. Combination therapy with lasers and topical or oral therapies have also shown to exhibit higher cumulative complete cure rates than any therapy alone [1,130–133]. Laser treatment is usually not covered, and the cost of laser treatments for onychomycosis can range from $400.00 to $1200.00 per session [126,129,134].

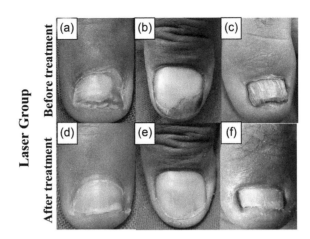

FIGURE 8.2
Pre- and post-treatment of onychomycosis with Q-Switched Nd:YAG (1064 nm) laser [137]. (a–c) Pre-treatment. (d–f) 3 months post-treatment with >75% clinical improvement. (From ref. [137] under Creative Commons licence.)

8.21 Nail Avulsion

Surgical nail avulsion is no longer commonly practised as treatment for onychomycosis due to low success rates, postoperative pain, risks of infection and shorter nail bed. Nail avulsion can be done when it is combined with antifungals and when there is single nail involvement [135,136]. Topical nail avulsion can also be performed with urea; however, this has a low success rate, although efficacy can be improved with topical antifungals [135,136].

8.22 Conclusion

When it comes to choosing the most appropriate treatment for a patient, one must consider various factors, including age, comorbidities, presence of mixed infections and concomitant medications. It is also important to note that there are various nail diseases such as psoriasis and lichen planus where secondary onychomycosis may be present where it is important to treat onychomycosis prior to starting patients on any immunosuppressive therapy.

References

1. Christenson JK, Peterson GM, Naunton M, et al. Challenges and opportunities in the management of onychomycosis. *J Fungi*. 2018;4(3):87.
2. Tosti A, Elewski BE. Onychomycosis: practical approaches to minimize relapse and recurrence. *Ski Appendage Disord*. 2016;2(1-2):83–7.
3. Bolognia JL, Schaffer JV, Serroni L, eds, Nail Disorders. *Dermatology*, 4th edition. Elsevier, 2017.

4. Lipner SR, Joseph WS, Vlahovic TC, et al. Therapeutic recommendations for the treatment of toenail onychomycosis in the US. *J Drugs Dermatol* 2021;20(10):1076–84.

5. Falotico JM, Lipner SR. Updated perspectives on the diagnosis and management of onychomycosis. *Clin, Cosmet Investig Dermatol*. 2022;15:1933–57.

6. Shoham S, Groll AH, Walsh TJ. Chapter 149: Antifungal Agents. In: Cohen J, Powderly W, Opal S, eds, *Infectious Diseases*, 3rd edition. Elsevier, 2010;1477–89.

7. Gupta AK. Ciclopirox nail lacquer topical solution 8%. *Ski Ther Lett*. 2000;6(1):1–5.

8. Ciclopirox FDA Label [Internet]. [cited 2023 Jul 26]. Available from: https://www.accessdata.fda.gov/drugsatfda_docs/label/2004/21022s004lbl.pdf

9. Kruk ME, Schwalbe N. The relation between intermittent dosing and adherence: preliminary insights. *Clin Ther*. 2006;28(12):1989–95.

10. Foley K, Gupta AK, Versteeg S, et al. Topical and device-based treatments for fungal infections of the toenails. *Cochrane Database Syst Rev*. 2020;1(1):CD012093.

11. Lipner SR, Scher RK. Onychomycosis treatment and prevention of recurrence. *J Am Acad Dermatol*. 2019;80(4):853–67.

12. Lipner SR, Scher RK, Rubin AI. Routine and Emerging Techniques in Onychomycosis Diagnosis. *Onychomycosis*. 2018;47–59.

13. Monti D, Mazzantini D, Tampucci S, et al. Ciclopirox and efinaconazole transungual permeation, antifungal activity, and proficiency to induce resistance in *Trichophyton rubrum*. *Antimicrob Agents Chemother*. 2019;63(10):e00442–19.

14. Groll AH, Piscitelli SC, Walsh TJ. Clinical pharmacology of systemic antifungal agents: a comprehensive review of agents in clinical use, current investigational compounds, and putative targets for antifungal drug development. *Adv Pharmacol*. 1998;44:343–500.

15. Warnock DW. Section 2: agents – antifungal agents. In: Finch RG, Greenwood D, Ragnar Norrby D, Whitley RJ, eds, *Antibiotic and Chemotherapy*, 9th edition. Elsevier Health Sciences, 2010;366–82. https://doi.org/10.1016/B978-0-7020-4064-1.00032-4.

16. Lipner SR, Scher Rk. Onychomycosis: topical therapy and devices. In: Rubin AJ et al., eds, *Scher and Daniel's Nails, Diagnosis, Surgery, Therapy*, 4th edition. Springer, 2018;173–83.

17. Blume-Peytavi U, Tosti A, Falqués M, et al. A multicentre, randomised, parallel-group, double-blind, vehicle-controlled and open-label, active-controlled study (versus amorolfine 5%), to evaluate the efficacy and safety of terbinafine 10% nail lacquer in the treatment of onychomycosis. *Mycoses*. 2022;65(4):392–401.

18. Banerjee M, Ghosh AK, Basak S, et al. Comparative evaluation of effectivity and safety of topical amorolfinr and clotrimazole in the treatment of Tinea corporis. *Indian J Dermatol*. 2011;56(6):657–62.

19. Reinel D. Topical treatment of onychomycosis with amorolfine 5% nail lacquer: comparative efficacy and tolerability of once and twice weekly use. *Dermatology*. 1992;184(Suppl 1):21–4.

20. Wang C, Canavan T, Elewski B. Topical therapies for onychomycosis. In: Rigopoulos D, Elewski B, Richert B, eds, *Onychomycosis: Diagnosis and Effective Management*. Wiley; 2018.

21. Amorolfine 5% Nail Lacquer Package Leaflet [Internet]. [cited 2023 Jul 28]. Available from: https://www.medicines.org.uk/emc/files/pil.8053.pdf

22. Marty JL, Lambert J, Jäckel A, et al. Treatment costs of three nail lacquers used in onychomycosis. *J Dermatol Treat*. 2005;16(5–6):299–307.

23. Kerydin (tavaborole) FDA Label [Internet]. [cited 2023 Jul 27]. Available from: https://www.accessdata.fda.gov/drugsatfda_docs/label/2018/204427s006lbl.pdf

24. Sharma N, Sharma D. An upcoming drug for onychomycosis: tavaborole. *J Pharmacol Pharmacother*. 2015;6(4):236–9.

25. Brody T. *Clinical trials*, Second Edition. Academic Press; 2016, pp. 483–568.

26. Gupta AK, Mays RR, Foley KA. Chapter 42: Topical Antifungal Agents. *Comprehensive Dermatologic Drug Therapy*(4th Edition), Elsevier, Indiana, USA. 2021;480–492. https://doi.org/10.1016/C2014-1-02097-2\.

27. Hui X, Baker SJ, Wester RC, et al. In Vitro penetration of a novel oxaborole antifungal (AN2690) into the human nail plate. *J Pharm Sci*. 2007;96(10):2622–31.

28. Elewski BE, Tosti A. Tavaborole for the treatment of onychomycosis. *Expert Opin Pharmacother*. 2014;15(10):1439–48.

29. Jinna S, Finch J. Spotlight on tavaborole for the treatment of onychomycosis. *Drug Des, Dev Ther.* 2015;9:6185–90.

30. Bill of the Month: $1,496 Kerydin Prescription Was a Costly Surprise: Shots – Health News: NPR [Internet]. [cited 2023 Jul 27]. Available from: https://www.npr.org/sections/health-sh ots/2018/03/16/594031602/financial-side-effects-from-a-prescription-for-toenail-fungus

31. Vlahovic TC. New Topical Antifungals. In: Tosti A, Vlahovic TC, Arenas R, editors, *Onychomycosis, An Illustrated Guide to Diagnosis and Treatment.* Springer Cham, Switzerland. 2017 pp. 197–203.

32. JUBLIA (efinaconazole) label [Internet]. [cited 2023 Jul 27]. Available from: https://www.accessdata.fda.gov/drugsatfda_docs/label/2014/203567s000lbl.pdf

33. Wang C, Cantrell W, Canavan T et al. Successful treatment of dermatophytomas in 19 patients using efinaconazole 10% solution. *Ski Appendage Disord.* 2019;5(5):304–8.

34. Lipner SR, Scher RK. Efinaconazole in the treatment of onychomycosis. *Infect Drug Resist.* 2015;8:163–72.

35. Wiederhold NP, Fothergill AW, McCarthy DI, et al. Luliconazole demonstrates potent in vitro activity against dermatophytes recovered from patients with onychomycosis. *Antimicrob Agents Chemother.* 2014;58(6):3553–5.

36. Watanabe S, Kishida H, Okubo A. Efficacy and safety of luliconazole 5% nail solution for the treatment of onychomycosis: a multicenter, double-blind, randomized phase III study. *J Dermatol.* 2017;44(7):753–9.

37. Gupta AK, Daigle D. A critical appraisal of once-daily topical luliconazole for the treatment of superficial fungal infections. *Infect Drug Resist.* 2016;9:1–6.

38. Gupta AK, Venkataraman M, Shear NH, et al. Onychomycosis in children – review on treatment and management strategies. *J Dermatol Treat.* 2022;33(3):1213–24.

39. Gupta AK, Talukder M, Venkataraman M. Review of the alternative therapies for onychomycosis and superficial fungal infections: posaconazole, fosravuconazole, voriconazole, otesec-onazole. *Int J Dermatol.* 2022;61(12):1431–41.

40. Eichenfield LF, Elewski B, Sugarman JL, et al. Safety, pharmacokinetics, and efficacy of efi-naconazole 10% topical solution for onychomycosis treatment in pediatric patients. *J drugs Dermatol: JDD.* 2020;19(9):867–72.

41. Rich P, Spellman M, Purohit V, et al. Tavaborole 5% topical solution for the treatment of toenail onychomycosis in pediatric patients: results from a phase 4 open-label study. *J Drugs Dermatol: JDD.* 2019;18(2):190–5.

42. Friedlander SF, Chan YC, Chan YH, et al. Onychomycosis does not always require systemic treatment for cure: a trial using topical therapy. *Pediatr Dermatol.* 2013;30(3):316–22.

43. Elewski BE, Aly R, Baldwin SL, et al. Efficacy and safety of tavaborole topical solution, 5%, a novel boron-based antifungal agent, for the treatment of toenail onychomycosis: results from 2 randomized phase-III studies. *J Am Acad Dermatol.* 2015;73(1):62–9.

44. Elewski BE, Rich P, Pollak R, et al. Efinaconazole 10% solution in the treatment of toenail ony-chomycosis: two phase III multicenter, randomized, double-blind studies. *J Am Acad Dermatol.* 2013;68(4):600–8.

45. Derby R, Rohal P, Jackson C, et al. Novel treatment of onychomycosis using over-the-counter mentholated ointment: a clinical case series. *J Am Board Fam Med.* 2011;24(1):69–74.

46. Buck DS, Nidorf DM, Addino JG. Comparison of two topical preparations for the treatment of onychomycosis: *Melaleuca alternifolia* (tea tree) oil and clotrimazole. *J Fam Pr.* 1994;38(6):601–5.

47. Syed TA, Qureshi ZA, Ali SM, et al. Treatment of toenail onychomycosis with 2% butenafine and 5% *Melaleuca alternifolia* (tea tree) oil in cream. *Trop Med Int Heal.* 1999;4(4):284–7.

48. Parekh M, Ramaiah G, Pashilkar P, et al. A pilot single centre, double blind, placebo controlled, randomized, parallel study of Calmagen(r) dermaceutical cream and lotion for the topical treatment of tinea and onychomycosis. *BMC Complement Altern Med.* 2017;17(1):464.

49. Menéndez S, Falcón L, Simón DR, et al. Efficacy of ozonized sunflower oil in the treatment of tinea pedis. *Mycoses.* 2002;45(7–8):329–32.

50. Sipponen P, Sipponen A, Lohi J, et al. Natural coniferous resin lacquer in treatment of toenail onychomycosis: an observational study. *Mycoses.* 2013;56(3):289–96.

51. Auvinen T, Tiihonen R, Soini M, et al. Efficacy of topical resin lacquer, amorolfine and oral terbinafine for treating toenail onychomycosis: a prospective, randomized, controlled, investigator-blinded, parallel-group clinical trial. *Br J Dermatol.* 2015;173(4):940–8.

52. Alessandrini A, Starace M, Bruni F, et al. An open study to evaluate effectiveness and tolerability of a nail oil composed of vitamin e and essential oils in mild to moderate distal subungual onychomycosis. *Ski Appendage Disord.* 2020;6(1):14–18.

53. Goldsmith S. Vitamin E and onychomycosis. *J Am Acad Dermatol.* 1983;8(6):910–1.

54. Darkes MJM, Scott LJ, Goa KL. Terbinafine. *Am J Clin Dermatol.* 2003;4(1):39–65.

55. Kreijkamp-Kaspers S, Hawke K, Guo L, et al. Oral antifungal medication for toenail onychomycosis. *Cochrane Database Syst Rev.* 2017;2017(7):CD010031.

56. RYDER NS. The mechanism of action of terbinafine. *Clin Exp Dermatol.* 1989;14(2):98–100.

57. Leyden J. Pharmacokinetics and pharmacology of terbinafine and itraconazole. *J Am Acad Dermatol.* 1998;38(5):S42–7.

58. Maddy AJ, Tosti A. In: Tosti A, Vlahovic TC, Arenas R, editors. *Onychomycosis.* Springer, Oxford, United Kingdom; 2018. pp. 118–22.

59. FDA. Food and Drug Administration. [cited 2023 Jul 25]. Lamisil (terbinafine hydroloride) tablets FDA label. Available from: https://www.accessdata.fda.gov/drugsatfda_docs/label/2012/020539s021lbl.pdf

60. Bermudez NM, Rodríguez-Tamez G, et al. Onychomycosis: old and new. *J Fungi.* 2023;9(5):559.

61. Iorizzo M, Piraccini BM, Tosti A. Today's treatments options for onychomycosis. *J Dtsch Dermatol Ges.* 2010;8(11):875–9.

62. Tosti A, Piraccini BM, Stinchi C, et al. Treatment of dermatophyte nail infections: an open randomized study comparing intermittent terbinafine therapy with continuous terbinafine treatment and intermittent itraconazole therapy. *J Am Acad Dermatol.* 1996;34(4):595–600.

63. Novartis. Novartis Lamisil Information [Internet]. [cited 2023 Jul 25]. Available from: https://www.novartis.com/sg-en/sites/novartis_sg/files/Lamisil-Jan2021.SIN-App190721.pdf

64. Akiyoshi T, Ishiuchi M, Imaoka A, et al. Variation in the inhibitory potency of terbinafine among genetic variants of CYP2D6. *Drug Metab Pharmacokinet.* 2015;30(4):321–4.

65. Abdel-Rahman SM, Gotschall RR, Kauffman RE, et al. Investigation of terbinafine as a CYP2D6 inhibitor in vivo. *Clin Pharmacol Ther.* 1999;65(5):465–72.

66. Dürrbeck A, Nenoff P. Terbinafin. *Hautarzt.* 2016;67(9):718–23.

67. Pollack A, Oliver M. Congenital glaucoma and incomplete congenital glaucoma in two siblings. *Acta Ophthalmol.* 1984;62(3):359–63.

68. Gupta AK, Ryder JE, Johnson AM. Cumulative meta-analysis of systemic antifungal agents for the treatment of onychomycosis. *Br J Dermatol.* 2004;150(3):537–44.

69. Sigurgeirsson B, Ólafsson JH, Steinsson JP, et al. Long-term effectiveness of treatment with terbinafine vs itraconazole in onychomycosis: a 5-year blinded prospective follow-up study. *Arch Dermatol.* 2002;138(3):353–7.

70. Havu V, Heikkilä H, Kuokkanen K, et al. A double-blind, randomized study to compare the efficacy and safety of terbinafine (Lamisil(r)) with fluconazole (Diflucan(r)) in the treatment of onychomycosis. *Br J Dermatol.* 2000;142(1):97–102.

71. Beule KD, Gestel JV. Pharmacology of Itraconazole. *Drugs.* 2001;61(Suppl 1):27–37.

72. Itraconazole FDA Label [Internet]. [cited 2023 Jul 29]. Available from: https://www.accessdata.fda.gov/drugsatfda_docs/label/2010/022484s000lbl.pdf

73. Sporanox (Itraconazole) FDA Label [Internet]. [cited 2023 Jul 29]. Available from: https://www.accessdata.fda.gov/drugsatfda_docs/label/2012/020083s048s049s050lbl.pdf

74. Sá DC de, Lamas APB, Tosti A. Oral therapy for onychomycosis: an evidence-based review. *Am J Clin Dermatol.* 2014;15(1):17–36.

75. Moreno-Coutiño G, Arenas R. Chapter 22: New Topical and Systemic Antifungals. In: Tosti A, Vlahovic TC, Arenas R, eds, *Onychomycosis, An Illustrated Guide to Diagnosis and Treatment.* Springer Cham, Switzerland; 2017. pp. 205–13.

76. Lohitnavy M, Lohitnavy O, Thangkeattiyanon O, et al. Reduced oral itraconazole bioavailability by antacid suspension. *J Clin Pharm Ther.* 2005;30(3):201–6.

77. Okuyan H, Altın C. Heart failure induced by itraconazole. *Indian J Pharmacol.* 2013;45(5):524–5.

78. Fung SL, Chau CH, Yew WW. Cardiovascular adverse effects during itraconazole therapy. *Eur Respir J.* 2008;32(1):240.

79. Gupta AK, Chwetzoff E, Rosso JD, et al. Hepatic safety of itraconazole. *J Cutan Med Surg: Inc Méd Surg Dermatol.* 2002;6(3):210–13.

80. Winston JA, Miller JL. Treatment of onychomycosis in diabetic patients. *Clin Diabetes.* 2006;24(4):160–6.

81. Boelaert J, Schurgers M, Matthys E, et al. Itraconazole pharmacokinetics in patients with renal dysfunction. *Antimicrob Agents Chemother.* 1988;32(10):1595–7.

82. Sigurgeirsson B. Systemic Therapy of Onychomycosis. In: Rubin A, et al., eds, *Scher and Daniel's Nails, Diagnosis, Surgery, Therapy*, 4th ed. Springer Cham, Philadelphia, PA, USA; 2018, pp. 185–214.

83. Tucker RM, Haq Y, Denning DW, et al. Adverse events associated with itraconazole in 189 patients on chronic therapy. *J Antimicrob Chemother.* 1990;26(4):561–6.

84. Diflucan (fluconazale) tablets label [Internet]. [cited 2023 Jul 30]. Available from: https://www.accessdata.fda.gov/drugsatfda_docs/label/2011/019949s051lbl.pdf

85. Skillman JJ, Paras C, Rosen M, et al. Improving cost efficiency on a vascular surgery service. *Am J Surg.* 2000;179(3):197–200.

86. Rosen T, Stein Gold LF. Antifungal drugs for onychomycosis: efficacy, safety, and mechanisms of action. *Semin Cutan Med Surg.* 2016;35(3S):S51–5.

87. Gupta AK, Drummond-Main C, Paquet M. Evidence-based optimal fluconazole dosing regimen for onychomycosis treatment. *J Dermatol Treat.* 2013;24(1):75–80.

88. Scher RK, Breneman D, Rich P, et al. Once-weekly fluconazole (150, 300, or 450 mg) in the treatment of distal subungual onychomycosis of the toenail. *J Am Acad Dermatol.* 1998;38(6):S77–86.

89. Ling MR, Swinyer LJ, Jarratt MT, et al. Once-weekly fluconazole (450 mg) for 4, 6, or 9 months of treatment for distal subungual onychomycosis of the toenail. *J Am Acad Dermatol.* 1998;38(6):S95–102.

90. Brown SJ. Efficacy of fluconazole for the treatment of onychomycosis. *Ann Pharmacother.* 2009;43(10):1684–91.

91. Arca E, Taştan HB, Akar A, et al. An open, randomized, comparative study of oral fluconazole, itraconazole and terbinafine therapy in onychomycosis. *J Dermatol Treat.* 2002;13(1):3–9.

92. Gupta AK, Gregurek-Novak T. Efficacy of itraconazole, terbinafine, fluconazole, griseofulvin and ketoconazole in the treatment of *Scopulariopsis brevicaulis* causing onychomycosis of the toes. *Dermatology.* 2001;202(3):235–8.

93. Lamisil (Terbinafine) FDA Package Insert [Internet]. [cited 2023 Aug 29]. Available from: https://www.accessdata.fda.gov/drugsatfda_docs/label/2019/020539s033lbl.pdf

94. Diflucan (Fluconazole) FDA Label [Internet]. [cited 2023 Aug 29]. Available from: https://www.accessdata.fda.gov/drugsatfda_docs/label/2019/019949s065,020090s047lbl.pdf

95. Thomas J, Jacobson GA, Narkowicz CK, et al. Toenail onychomycosis: an important global disease burden. *J Clin Pharm Ther.* 2010;35(5):497–519.

96. Leung AKC, Lam JM, Leong KF, et al. Onychomycosis: an updated review. *Inflamm Allergy - Drug Targets.* 2019;14(1):32–45.

97. Ishida K, de Morais Barroso V. Allylamines, morpholine derivatives, fluoropyrimidines, and griseofulvin. In: Zaragoza O, editor. *Encyclopedia of Mycology.* Cambridge, MA: Elsevier; 2021. pp. 449–55.

98. Griseofulvin FDA Label [Internet]. [cited 2023 Jul 30]. Available from: https://www.accessdata.fda.gov/drugsatfda_docs/label/2016/050475s057lbl.pdf

99. Gupta AK, Cooper EA, Lynde CW. The efficacy and safety of terbinafine in children. *Dermatol Clin.* 2003;21(3):511–20.

100. Gupta AK, Mays RR, Versteeg SG, et al. Onychomycosis in children: safety and efficacy of antifungal agents. *Pediatr Dermatol.* 2018;35(5):552–9.

101. Chen S, Sun KY, Feng XW, et al. Efficacy and safety of itraconazole use in infants. *World J Pediatr.* 2016;12(4):399–407.

102. Wang Y, Lipner SR. Analysis of utilization, cost and, prescription trends of onychomycosis medications among Medicare patients. *J Am Acad Dermatol.* 2022;86(2):440–2.

103. Stolmeier DA, Stratman HB, McIntee TJ, et al. Utility of laboratory test result monitoring in patients taking oral terbinafine or griseofulvin for dermatophyte infections. *JAMA Dermatol.* 2018;154(12):1409.

104. Homer K, Robson J, Solaiman S, et al. Reducing liver function tests for statin monitoring: an observational comparison of two clinical commissioning groups. *Br J Gen Pr.* 2017;67(656):e194–200.

105. Muddasani S, Housholder A, Fleischer AB. The cost of liver function tests for terbinafine: an unnecessary expense. *J Dermatol Treat.* 2022;33(3):1789.

106. Gupta A, Baran R, Summerbell R. Onychomycosis: strategies to improve efficacy and reduce recurrence. *J Eur Acad Dermatol Venereol.* 2002;16(6):579–86.

107. Sigurgeirsson B, Paul C, Curran D, et al. Prognostic factors of mycological cure following treatment of onychomycosis with oral antifungal agents. *Br J Dermatol.* 2002;147(6):1241–3.

108. Gupta AK, Konnikov N, Lynde CW. Single-blind, randomized, prospective study on terbinafine and itraconazole for treatment of dermatophyte toenail onychomycosis in the elderly. *J Am Acad Dermatol.* 2001;44(3):479–84.

109. Fungal Nail Infections | Fungal Diseases | CDC [Internet]. [cited 2023 Jul 26]. Available from: https://www.cdc.gov/ringworm/hcp/clinical-overview/index.html

110. FDA. Noxafil (Posaconazole) Label [Internet]. [cited 2023 Jul 25]. Available from: https://www.accessdata.fda.gov/drugsatfda_docs/label/2015/022003s018s020,0205053s002s004,0205596s001s003lbl.pdf

111. Greer ND. Posaconazole (Noxafil): a new triazole antifungal agent. *Bayl Univ Méd Cent Proc.* 2007;20(2):188–96.

112. Spencer R, Curran S, Musa S. Hypnosedatives and anxiolytics. In: Aronson JK, editor, *Side Effects of Drugs Annual.* Elsevier, New York, NY, USA; 2011; 33, pp. 71–88.

113. Groll AH, Walsh TJ. *Feigin and Cherry's Textbook of Pediatric Infectious Diseases,* 6th ed., Elsevier; 2009. pp. 3271–308.

114. Elewski B, Pollak R, Ashton S, et al A. A randomized, placebo- and active-controlled, parallel-group, multicentre, investigator-blinded study of four treatment regimens of posaconazole in adults with toenail onychomycosis. *Br J Dermatol.* 2012;166(2):389–98.

115. Oral Antifungal Agent Nailin(r) Capsules Approved in Japan; News Release, 2018, Eisai Co., Ltd. [Internet]. [cited 2023 Jul 25]. Available from: https://www.eisai.com/news/2018/news201806.html

116. Inoue T, Watabe D, Tsunemi Y, et al. Outcome of fosravuconazole treatment for onychomycosis refractory to topical antifungal agents. *J Dermatol.* 2023; 50(8):1014–1019.

117. Watanabe S, Tsubouchi I, Okubo A. Efficacy and safety of fosravuconazole L-lysine ethanolate, a novel oral triazole antifungal agent, for the treatment of onychomycosis: a multicenter, double-blind, randomized phase III study. *J Dermatol.* 2018;45(10):1151–9.

118. FDA. VFEND (Voriconazole) FDA Label [Internet]. [cited 2023 Jul 25]. Available from: https://www.accessdata.fda.gov/drugsatfda_docs/label/2019/021266s039,021267s050,021630s029lbl.pdf

119. Nofal A, Fawzy MM, El-Hawary EE. Successful treatment of resistant onychomycosis with voriconazole in a liver transplant patient. *Dermatol Ther.* 2020;33(6):e14014.

120. Chang CC, Slavin MA. Albaconazole. *Kucers' The Use of Antibiotics, A Clinical Review of Antibacterial, Antifungal, Antiparasitic, and Antiviral Drugs,* 7th ed. CRC Press, Boca Raton, FL; 2018. pp. 2870–5.

121. Sigurgeirsson B, Rossem K van, Malahias S, et al. A phase II, randomized, double-blind, placebo-controlled, parallel group, dose-ranging study to investigate the efficacy and safety of 4 dose regimens of oral albaconazole in patients with distal subungual onychomycosis. *J Am Acad Dermatol.* 2013;69(3):416–425.e1.

122. VIVJOA (oteseconazole) FDA Label [Internet]. [cited 2023 Jul 26]. Available from: https://www.accessdata.fda.gov/drugsatfda_docs/label/2022/215888s000lbl.pdf

123. Hoy SM. Oteseconazole: first approval. *Drugs.* 2022;82(9):1017–23.

124. Elewski B, Brand S, Degenhardt T, et al. A phase II, randomized, double-blind, placebo-controlled, dose-ranging study to evaluate the efficacy and safety of VT-1161 oral tablets in the treatment of patients with distal and lateral subungual onychomycosis of the toenail*. *Br J Dermatol.* 2021;184(2):270–80.

125. FDA, medical devices and clinical trial design for the treatment or improvement in the appearance of fungally infected nails: guidance for industry and food and drug administration staff. [Internet].[cited 2023 Jul 26]. Available from: https://www.fda.gov/files/medical%20devices/published/Medical-Devices-and-Clinical-Trial-Design-for-the-Treatment-or-Improvement-in-the-Appearance-of-Fungally-Infected-Nails---Guidance-for-Industry-and-Food-and-Drug-Administration-Staff.pdf

126. Gupta AK, Versteeg SG. A critical review of improvement rates for laser therapy used to treat toenail onychomycosis. *J Eur Acad Dermatol Venereol.* 2017;31(7):1111–18.

127. Critical review of improvement rates in onychomycosis patients treated with laser therapy. *J Am Acad Dermatol.* 2017;76(6):AB86.

128. Gupta AK, Simpson FC. Laser Therapy for Onychomycosis. *J Cutan Med Surg.* 2013;17(5):301–7.

129. Ma W, Si C, Carrero LMK, et al. Laser treatment for onychomycosis. *Medicine.* 2019;98(48):e17948.

130. Zhang J, Lu S, Huang H, et al. Combination therapy for onychomycosis using a fractional 2940-nm Er:YAG laser and 5% amorolfine lacquer. *Lasers Méd Sci.* 2016;31(7):1391–6.

131. Park KY, Suh JH, Kim BJ, et al. Randomized clinical trial to evaluate the efficacy and safety of combination therapy with short-pulsed 1,064-nm neodymium-doped yttrium aluminium garnet laser and amorolfine nail lacquer for onychomycosis. *Ann Dermatol.* 2017;29(6):699–705.

132. Lim EH, Kim HR, Park YO, et al. Toenail onychomycosis treated with a fractional carbon-dioxide laser and topical antifungal cream. *J Am Acad Dermatol.* 2014;70(5):918–23.

133. Xu Y, Miao X, Zhou B, et al. Combined oral terbinafine and long-pulsed 1,064-nm Nd. *Dermatol Surg.* 2014;40(11):1201–7.

134. Hollmig ST, Rahman Z, Henderson MT, et al. Lack of efficacy with 1064-nm neodymium:yttrium-aluminum-garnet laser for the treatment of onychomycosis: a randomized, controlled trial. *J Am Acad Dermatol.* 2014;70(5):911–17.

135. Grover C, Bansal S, Nanda S, et al. Combination of surgical avulsion and topical therapy for single nail onychomycosis: a randomized controlled trial. *Br J Dermatol.* 2007;157(2):364–8.

136. Grover C, Khurana A, Jain R, et al. Transungual surgical excision of subungual glomus tumour. *J Cutan Aesthetic Surg.* 2013;6(4):196–203.

137. Nasif GA, Amin AA, Ragaie MH. Q-switched Nd:YAG laser versus itraconazole pulse therapy in treatment of onychomycosis: a clinical dermoscopic and mycologic study. *J Cosmet Dermatol.* 2023;22(6):1757–63.

138. Gupta AK, Fleckman P, Baran R. Ciclopirox nail lacquer topical solution 8% in the treatment of toenail onychomycosis. *J Am Acad Dermatol.* 2000;43(4):S70–80.

139. Sigurgeirsson B, Steingrímsson Ó. Risk factors associated with onychomycosis. *J Eur Acad Dermatol Venereol.* 2004;18(1):48–51.

140. Gupta A, Chang P, Rosso JD, et al. Onychomycosis in children: prevalence and management. *Pediatr Dermatol.* 1998;15(6):464–71.

141. Gupta AK, Sibbald RG, Lynde CW, et al. Onychomycosis in children: prevalence and treatment strategies. *J Am Acad Dermatol.* 1997;36(3):395–402.

142. Ameen M, Lear JT, Madan V, et al. British association of dermatologists' guidelines for the management of onychomycosis 2014. *Br J Dermatol.* 2014;171(5):937–58.

143. Gupta AK, Cooper EA, Ginter G. Efficacy and safety of itraconazole use in children. *Dermatol Clin.* 2003;21(3):521–35.

144. Gupta AK, Venkataraman M, Shear NH, et al. Labeled use of efinaconazole topical solution 10% in treating onychomycosis in children and a review of the management of pediatric onychomycosis. *Dermatol Ther.* 2020;33(4):e13613.

145. Krishna G, Ma L, Martinho M, et al. Determination of posaconazole levels in toenails of adults with onychomycosis following oral treatment with four regimens of posaconazole for 12 or 24 weeks. *Antimicrob Agents Chemother.* 2011;55(9):4424–6.

146. Dietz AJ, Barnard JC, Rossem K van. A randomized, double-blind, multiple-dose, placebo-controlled, dose escalation study with a 3-cohort parallel group design to investigate the tolerability and pharmacokinetics of albaconazole in healthy subjects. *Clin Pharmacol Drug Dev.* 2014;3(1):25–33.

9

New and Emerging Therapies for the Nail

Shari Lipner and Jade Conway

9.1 Novel Oral Therapies

Traditionally, systemic oral medications for onychomycosis treatment, including terbinafine or triazoles (itraconazole, fluconazole), have generally been preferred over topical antifungal agents due to their accessibility, shorter courses and efficacy. Risks for oral medications include drug–drug interactions and adverse systemic side effects [1]. Novel oral therapies for onychomycosis show promise as alternatives to current treatments.

Posaconazole is a triazole antifungal, chemically similar to itraconazole, and has potent activity against dermatophytes [2]. In a phase IIb, randomized, placebo- and active-controlled, multicentre trial, 218 adults with toenail onychomycosis received one of six treatments: posaconazole (oral suspension) 100, 200 or 400 mg once daily for 24 weeks, posaconazole 400 mg once daily for 12 weeks, oral terbinafine 250 mg tablets once daily for 12 weeks or placebo for 24 weeks [3]. Compared to placebo, all posaconazole treatments had significantly higher proportions of patients with complete cure rates at 48 weeks ($p < 0.012$). Patients receiving posaconazole 200 and 400 mg for 24 weeks had higher complete cure rates (54.1% and 45.5%, respectively) vs. patients receiving terbinafine (37%), although differences were not statistically significant. Patients receiving posaconazole 400 mg for 12 weeks showed lower complete cure rates (20%). Patients who received posaconazole 200 and 400 mg for 24 weeks showed similar mycologic cure rates (70.3% and 78.8%, respectively) compared to patients who received terbinafine (71.4%) [3]. Posaconazole was well-tolerated and showed a good safety profile [3,4].

Albaconazole is a broad-spectrum azole antifungal with activity against dermatophytes, yeasts and other non-dermatophyte filamentous fungi. Since it has an average half-life of 70.5 hours after a single oral dose, it may allow for weekly dosing for treatment of onychomycosis [5]. In a phase II, double-blind, placebo-controlled, multicentre study, 582 adults with distal subungual onychomycosis affecting at least one great toenail were assigned to one of five treatment regimens: 100, 200 or 400 mg albaconazole capsules once-weekly for 36 weeks, 400 mg albaconazole capsules once-weekly for 24 weeks plus 12 weeks placebo, or placebo capsules for 36 weeks [5]. The primary endpoint was proportion of patients achieving effective treatment, defined as mycologic cure with clear/almost clear nail (<10% of nail plate affected). Compared to placebo (1%), all treatment groups achieved greater effective treatment rates at week 52 ($p < 0.001$). Efficacy increased with higher doses: 54% (400 mg, 36 weeks), 38% (400 mg, 24 weeks), 39% (200 mg, 36 weeks), 21% (100 mg, 36 weeks). Clinical, mycologic and complete cure rates increased in a dose-dependent manner (16%–34%, 34%–71% and 12%–33%, respectively) and were higher in all treatment groups

DOI: 10.1201/9781003381648-10

compared to placebo ($p<0.001$) [5]. Less than 3% of patients reported mild-to-moderate treatment-related adverse events.

Fosravuconazole L-lysine ethanolate (F-RVCZ) is an azole prodrug of ravuconazole, formulated to achieve greater bioavailability after oral administration compared to ravuconazole. It is approved for the treatment of onychomycosis in Japan (100 mg once daily for 12 weeks) [4,6]. In a phase III, randomized, double-blinded, multicentre study, 153 Japanese patients with toenail onychomycosis received treatment with either 100 mg F-RVCZ or placebo once daily for 12 weeks. At week 48, complete cure rate was higher for F-RVCZ than placebo (59.4% vs. 5.8%, $p<0.001$). Mycological cure rate at week 48 was higher with F-RVCZ than placebo (82% vs. 20%, $p<0.001$) [7]. No serious adverse drug reactions occurred [7].

A systematic review and meta-analysis of 40 randomized controlled clinical trials (9568 total patients) evaluated the effect of oral antifungals on mycological cure for treatment of toenail onychomycosis with ranking probabilities calculated by surface under the cumulative ranking curve (SUCRA) [8]. Albaconazole 400 mg was considered the more effective treatment for mycological cure (SUCRA 89.5%, OR 0.02 [95% CI 0.01–0.07] vs. placebo), followed by posaconazole 200 and 400 mg (SUCRA over 75%, OR 0.03 [95% CI 0.01–0.09] and OR 0.02 [95% CI 0.01–0.08], vs. placebo) and terbinafine 250 and 350 mg (SUCRA over 75%, OR 0.03 [95% CI 0.02–0.06] and OR 0.03 [95% CI 0.01–0.07], vs. placebo). While albaconazole, posaconazole and terbinafine were considered the most effective therapies for onychomycosis, itraconazole was considered the safest, based on rates of discontinuation due to adverse events [8].

Oteseconazole (VT-1161) is a tetrazole and novel inhibitor of the lanosterol demethylase (CYP51) enzyme, recently studied but not yet FDA approved for onychomycosis treatment [1,9]. In a phase II, randomized, double-blinded, placebo-controlled, multicentre study, 259 adult patients with distal or lateral subungual toenail onychomycosis with 25%–75% mycotic involvement received one of five regimens: 300 or 600 mg VT-1161 once daily for 2 weeks followed by a once-weekly dose for 10 or 22 weeks, or placebo [10]. Complete and mycologic cure rates were higher at week 60 in all treatment groups receiving VT-1161 (41%–45%, 65%–75%, respectively) compared to placebo (0%, 13%, respectively) ($p<0.001$) [10].

9.2 Non-oral Terbinafine Alternatives

Terbinafine is a well-known antifungal agent that non-competitively inhibits squalene epoxidase, a key enzyme involved in ergosterol biosynthesis, which is essential for fungal membrane integrity [11]. Oral terbinafine is one of the most commonly used drugs for onychomycosis treatment, but is associated with adverse events, drug–drug interactions and rising rates of treatment failure or recurrence [12]. Given these disadvantages with oral administration, non-oral terbinafine alternatives with less systemic effects are also being explored.

MOB-015 is a topical terbinafine 10% solution that has been studied for the treatment of mild-to-moderate toenail onychomycosis (Table 9.1). In a clinical trial evaluating the safety and efficacy of MOB-015, 365 patients aged 12–72 years with subungual onychomycosis affecting at least one great toenail were randomized to once-daily application of MOB-015 or matching inactive vehicle for 48 weeks, followed by 4 weeks of follow-up [12]. At week

TABLE 9.1

Summary of Clinical Trial Results for MOB-015 Topical Terbinafine Treatment

Study	Study Type	Study Participants	Intervention	Comparison	Outcome Measures	Relevant Results	Relevant Adverse Effects
Gupta et al.[11]	Randomized, double-blind, two-arm, parallel-group, multicentre clinical trial	365 patients with distal-lateral onychomycosis confirmed by culture	MOB-015 topical treatment once daily for 48 weeks (n = 246)	Matching inactive vehicle (urea, lactic acid, propylene glycol) topical treatment once daily for 48 weeks (n = 119)	Complete cure (mycological cure plus 0% clinical disease involvement) at 52 weeks; secondary outcomes included treatment success (mycological cure plus ≤10% clinical disease involvement of target toenail) at 52 weeks	4.5% and 0% of MOB-015 and vehicle patients, respectively, achieved complete cure ($p = 0.0195$) at 52 weeks; 69.9% and 27.7% of MOB-15 and vehicle patients, respectively, achieved mycologic cure at 52 weeks ($p < 0.001$); 15.4% and 4.2% of MOB-015 and vehicle patients, respectively, achieved treatment success ($p = 0.0018$)	Minor application site adverse effects in 0.4%–2.8% of MOB-015 and vehicle patients including contact dermatitis, erythema and nail plate bleeding
Blume-Peytavi et al.[12]	Randomized, double-blind, parallel-group, multicentre clinical trial	953 patients with mild-moderate distal lateral onychomycosis confirmed by KOH and culture	MOB-015 topical treatment once daily for 4 weeks, then once weekly for 44 weeks (n = 406)	Vehicle topical treatment once daily for 4 weeks then once weekly for 44 weeks (n = 410) or amorolfine 5% topical treatment once weekly for 48 weeks (n = 137)	Complete cure rate (negative KOH, negative culture and no residual clinical involvement) at 60 weeks; secondary outcomes included responder rate (mycological cure plus ≤10% clinical disease involvement of target toenail) at 60 weeks	5.67% of MOB-015 patients achieved complete cure compared to 2.2% of vehicle patients (OR = 2.68; 95% CI: 1.22–5.86, $p = 0.0138$) and 2.92% of amorolfine patients (OR = 2.00; 95% CI: 0.67–5.88, $p = 0.2095$) at 60 weeks; responder rate for MOB-015 patients was 6.65% compared to 3.14% of vehicle patients and 3.65% of amorolfine patients; MOB-015 patients had significantly higher responder rates ($p = 0.0377$) and mycological cure rates ($p = 0.0016$) compared with vehicle	1.89% of all patients reported adverse effects relating to "skin and subcutaneous tissue disorders"; only one patient in vehicle group showed evidence of finger irritation

52, mycological cure rate was higher with MOB-015 than vehicle (69.9% vs. 27.7%, $p < 0.001$) and complete cure rate was achieved in 4.5% vs. 0% of patients, respectively ($p = 0.0195$). The complete cure rate was low because while the vehicle enhances the ability of terbinafine to penetrate the nail plate, it increases nail opacity, thereby interfering with complete cure rate assessment [12]. Overall, 95.9% of MOB-015-treated patients had negative fungal cultures compared with 58% of vehicle-treated patients at 52 weeks [12]. No serious adverse events related to the study medication were reported [12]. In another clinical trial evaluating topical terbinafine 10% solution, 953 patients >12 years of age with subungual onychomycosis of at least one great toenail received treatment with topical terbinafine 10%, its vehicle or topical amorolfine 5% [11]. Topical terbinafine and its vehicle were administered once daily for 4 weeks then once-weekly for 44 weeks, and topical amorolfine 5% was administered once-weekly for 48 weeks with a 12-week follow-up. At week 60, complete cure rates for the terbinafine, vehicle and amorolfine groups were 5.67%, 2.20% and 2.92%, respectively. Patients treated with MOB-015 had significantly higher complete cure rates compared with vehicle ($p = 0.0138$) but not amorolfine ($p = 0.2095$). Topical terbinafine was well-tolerated with no systemic adverse reactions [11]. MOB-015 demonstrated excellent mycological cure rate without systemic adverse reactions or drug–drug interactions associated with oral formulations.

As topical formulations have typically demonstrated lower efficacy in treating onychomycosis compared to oral medications due to nail plate penetration, delivery approaches for optimizing drug penetration are being explored. TDT-067 is a carrier-based form of 15 mg/mL terbinafine in transfersome administered in a liquid spray. The lipid aggregates of the transfersome carrier are highly deformable with high surface hydrophilicity to ensure a high level of local drug accumulation unlike typical topical agents [13]. In a study comparing *in vitro* antifungal activity of TDT-067 with "naked" terbinafine (not in transfersome vesicles), TDT-067 had potent activity against dermatophyte strains with minimal inhibitory concentration (MIC) of 0.00003–0.015 mg/mL. Overall, TDT-067 MIC_{50} values were 8-fold lower than those of naked terbinafine (p value not reported), demonstrating better antifungal activity than the conventional terbinafine preparation [13].

Transungual (P-3058) and patch (HTU-520) delivery methods for terbinafine are being explored [14]. Use of polymer nanoparticles to enhance penetration into the nail plate is being studied in transungual terbinafine formulations [15]. Additionally, novel film-forming agents such as hydroxypropyl chitosan (HPCH) have been evaluated for use in transungual delivery of terbinafine solution [16]. Clinical trials to investigate these alternatives have been registered, but results are not yet published.

9.3 Novel Topical Agents

Until recently, topical onychomycosis treatment options were limited to ciclopirox 8% nail lacquer, amorolfine, efinaconazole and tavaborole [17]. Development of novel topical therapies has focused on formulation enhancements and efforts and broad-spectrum antifungal activity.

Due to the insoluble nature of their vehicles, use of ciclopirox 8% and amorolfine 5% requires nail filing with application. More recently, a new water-soluble ciclopirox 8% formulation in HPCH technology (P-3051) was developed. HPCH forms a film on the nail surface, allows for longer contact, and has better penetration and efficacy compared to traditional insoluble lacquers [18]. Lack of nail filing requirements and easy removal with water also contribute to greater patient compliance.

In a randomized, placebo-controlled, multicentre study comparing P-3051 to insoluble 8% ciclopirox nail lacquer, 467 patients with onychomycosis of at least one great toenail were assigned to receive daily application of P-3051, the reference lacquer or placebo for 48 weeks with a 12-week follow-up period [19]. At week 60, the complete cure rate for the P-3051 group was significantly higher than the reference ciclopirox 8% lacquer and placebo groups (12.7% vs. 5.8% vs. 1.3%, respectively; $p<0.05$) [19]. Local erythema and burning were three and four times more frequent, respectively, with the reference lacquer compared to P-3051, likely due to differences in inactive drug ingredients. In another randomized, double-blinded controlled study, 120 adult patients with toenail onychomycosis were treated for 48 weeks with either P-3051 daily or amorolfine 5% twice weekly. Patients treated with P-3051 showed higher complete cure rates compared to those treated with amorolfine (35.0% vs. 11.7%, respectively; $p<0.001$). At week 48, all patients treated with P-3051 achieved mycological cure compared to 81.7% of patients treated with amorolfine ($p<0.001$) [18].

To further enhance therapeutic efficacy of topical ciclopirox, a new water-soluble formulation was developed. Ciclopirox hydrolacquer (DexULac) uses a novel vehicle with Ciclo-Tech technology that contains a solubilizing agent (hydroxypropyl-β-cyclodextrin), a permeability-enhancing substance (sodium lauryl sulphate) and a film-forming agent (poloxamer 407) to enhance diffusion through the keratin surface of the nail and increase the concentration and permanence of the active ingredient compared to other lacquers [20]. In a phase III, randomized, double-blinded, multicentre clinical trial, 381 adult patients with distal onychomycosis affecting at least one great toenail were assigned to apply ciclopirox hydrolacquer, ciclopirox 8% lacquer in HPCH or vehicle once daily for 48 weeks with a follow-up period of 4 weeks [20]. At week 52, patients in the ciclopirox hydrolacquer group achieved higher mycological cure rate (based on both negative culture and potassium hydroxide preparation [KOH]) compared to HPCH lacquer and vehicle groups (32.0% vs. 27% vs. 23.3%, respectively, no p value reported). Negative culture rates were 47.2% vs. 46% vs. 34.4%, respectively, although only ciclopirox hydrolacquer demonstrated significant superiority vs. vehicle ($p=0.039$) [20]. These newer formulations of ciclopirox show better local safety profiles, have less bothersome application and removal procedures, compared to the older ciclopirox formulation.

Luliconazole is a novel, broad-spectrum imidazole antifungal originally developed in Japan that interferes with ergosterol biosynthesis through inhibition of sterol 14α-demethylase [9,21]. In a phase III, randomized, double-blind, multicentre study, 292 adult patients with onychomycosis of at least one great toenail were assigned to receive once-daily treatment of either luliconazole 5% solution or vehicle for 48 weeks [22]. At week 48, complete cure rate was higher in the luliconazole group vs. vehicle (14.9% vs. 5.1%, respectively; $p=0.012$). Additionally, 45.4% of patients treated with luliconazole had negative microscopy at week 48 compared to 31.2% of patients treated with vehicle ($p=0.026$). There were no serious adverse drug reactions [22].

ME1111 is a newer topical antifungal inhibiting mitochondrial electron transfer through inhibition of succinate dehydrogenase and leads to blockade of ATP production. It has *in vitro* antifungal activity against *Trichophyton rubrum* and *Trichophyton mentagrophytes*, and has small molecular weight which may make it penetrate nails efficiently [9,23]. *In vitro* studies demonstrated greater nail penetration of ME1111 compared to that of ciclopirox, efinaconazole and amorolfine. Toxicity studies have found no concerns about its safety profile [24–26]. A phase II randomized, double-blinded, vehicle-controlled study in patients with toenail onychomycosis (NCT02022215) has been completed, but results have not been published.

NP213 (NVXT, Novexatin) is a novel topical synthetic antimicrobial peptide under investigation for onychomycosis treatment. The positively charged peptide, consisting of seven arginine amino acids arranged in a hydrophilic cationic cyclic peptide, exerts its antifungal action by rapidly penetrating the negatively charged nail and evading the proteolytic activity of dermatophyte peptidases and proteases. It has both antifungal and sporicidal activity against *T. rubrum* by targeting the fungal cytoplasmic membrane [27,28]. Efficacy, safety and pharmacokinetics of NP213 were evaluated in two studies. In the first randomized, placebo-controlled trial, phase I enrolled 12 adult patients with toenail onychomycosis and phase IIa enrolled 48 adult patients with toenail onychomycosis. Patients in both phases received daily application of NP213 or vehicle (2:1 ratio) for 28 days with extended follow-up. Overall, 43.3% of patients treated with NP213 reported clinical improvement and had at least one negative culture over 180 days compared to 18.75% in vehicle-treated patients (*p* value not reported) [29]. The second phase IIa randomized, double-blinded, placebo-controlled pilot study enrolled 47 adult patients with toenail onychomycosis to receive daily application of either NP213 or placebo (3:1 ratio) for 28 days with longer follow-up. Overall, 56.5% of patients treated with NP213 were culture negative at 1 year, whereas none of the vehicle-treated patients were culture negative (*p* value not reported) [29]. NP213 has demonstrated good efficacy and biostability. Phase III trials are needed to expand data on efficacy.

9.4 Alternative Therapies

Laser-based devices are approved only for temporary cosmetic improvement of onychomycosis, not cure [30]. Lasers are thought to inhibit fungal growth by selective photothermolysis [31]. The short-pulsed and Q-switched Nd:YAG 1064-nm lasers are FDA approved for temporary cosmetic improvement of onychomycosis, and other lasers, including the carbon dioxide (CO_2) and diode laser, are in development [1]. Laser treatments may improve nail appearance; however, there is limited evidence on their ability to eradicate pathogenic fungi and maintain clinical clearance. Most studies to date have only focused on aesthetic endpoints and provided data on clinical improvement, but lack data on efficacy rates compared with traditional oral and topical treatments (Table 9.2).

In a review comparing improvement rates with lasers vs. FDA-approved traditional onychomycosis treatments, laser treatment ($n=2$ studies) was associated with lower mycologic cure rates (11%) compared to oral and topical therapies (29%–61%) [32]. In a retrospective study of 23 patients with mycologically confirmed onychomycosis of the great toenail treated with the Nd:YAG 1064 nm laser at variable intervals and assessed at week 12, 78% of patients showed temporary improvement in appearance of nails and 46% of patients showed decrease in nail involvement >50% from baseline; only two patients (9%) achieved clinical cure [30]. A systematic review with meta-analysis on available laser treatments for onychomycosis ($n=35$ studies, 1,723 patients, 4278 nails) showed an overall mycological cure rate of 63% (95% CI: 0.53–0.73) [31]. Mycological cure rate with the Nd:YAG 1064 nm laser was 63% (95% CI: 0.51–0.74) while mycological cure rate with CO_2 lasers was 74% (95% CI: 0.37–0.98). Adverse effects, such as pain and bleeding, are common [31].

TABLE 9.2

Summary of Clinical Trial Results for Laser, PDT and Plasma Therapy Treatments

Study	Study Type	Study Participants	Intervention	Comparison	Primary Outcome Measures	Relevant Results	Relevant Adverse Effects
Landsman et al.[33]	Randomized, single-blinded, controlled clinical trial	34 patients with mild-to-severe onychomycosis of toenails confirmed by culture and PAS, with 37 toes eligible for treatment	Treatment with Noveon dual-wavelength near-infrared diode laser on days 1, 14, 42 and 120 ($n = 26$)	Control "sham" laser treatment with no energy output on days 1, 14, 42 and 120 ($n = 11$)	Clinical improvement (measured by clear nail growth) and mycological cure at 180 days	85% of treated toenails showed clinical improvement at 180 days; 65.4% of treated toes and 9.1% of control toes showed at least 3 mm of clear nail growth at 180 days ($p = 0.0015$). 39% of treated toenails and 9.1% of control toes showed concurrent mycological cure at 180 days	Heat or tingling sensation during approximately 50% of treatments
Gilaberte et al.[37]	Randomized, controlled, multicentre clinical trial	40 patients with onychomycosis confirmed by culture	3 weekly treatment sessions of methyl aminolevulinate PDT (MAL-PDT) with urea 40% cream applied prior to treatments ($n = 22$)	3 weekly treatment sessions of placebo (red light) PDT (pPDT) with urea 40% cream applied prior to treatments ($n = 18$)	Clinical improvement scored with onychomycosis severity index (OSI) and mycological cure at 36 weeks	Mean differences in OSI were −11 (95% CI: −16.4 to −5.54) in the MAL-PDT group and −8 (95% CI: −13.6 to −2.36) in the pPDT group at 36 weeks; 18.18% of the MAL-PDT group and 5.56% of the pPDT group (95% CI: 2.98–9.69, $p = 0.23$) showed complete clinical improvement (OSI = 0) at 36 weeks; 31.82% of the MAL-PDT group and 11.11% of the pPDT group achieved mycological cure at 36 weeks	Pigmentation in 4.6% and inflammation in 18.2% of MAL-PDT patients

(Continued)

TABLE 9.2 (*Continued*)

Summary of Clinical Trial Results for Laser, PDT and Plasma Therapy Treatments

Study	Study Type	Study Participants	Intervention	Comparison	Primary Outcome Measures	Relevant Results	Relevant Adverse Effects
Souza et al.[38]	Open-label, controlled clinical trial	22 total patients: 11 patients with severe distal-lateral onychomycosis of toenails (group A) and 11 patients with mild-to-moderate distal-lateral onychomycosis of toenails (group B)	Group A treated with PDT with 2% methylene blue aqueous solution biweekly for 6 months	Group B treated with PDT with 2% methylene blue aqueous solution biweekly for 6 months	Clinical response at 48 weeks	63.6% and 100% of patients in groups A and B, respectively, achieved complete clinical response at 48 weeks. 36.4% of group A achieved marked clinical response at 48 weeks	None
Sobhy et al.[39]	Prospective, randomized clinical trial	51 patients with onychomycosis confirmed by culture	Group A: 6 bimonthly treatments of PDT with methylene blue 2% and intense pulsed light (IPL)	Group B: 6 bimonthly treatments of fractional CO_2 laser; Group C: 6 bimonthly treatments of fractional CO_2 laser (2 passes), followed by PDT	Clinical improvement (assessed by calculating increase in clear proximal nail plate diameter) and mycologic cure post-treatments	Mean increase of proximal nail diameter percentage after treatment was highest in group C (52.94 ± 20.24) vs. group B (43.82 ± 21.03) and group A (35.29 ± 17.0) ($p = 0.044$) post-treatments; mycological cure was highest in group C (88.2%) followed by group B (76.5%) and group A (64.7%) post-treatments	Mild-moderate pain and discoloration reported in all three groups

(*Continued*)

TABLE 9.2 (*Continued*)

Summary of Clinical Trial Results for Laser, PDT and Plasma Therapy Treatments

Study	Study Type	Study Participants	Intervention	Comparison	Primary Outcome Measures	Relevant Results	Relevant Adverse Effects
Lipner et al.[40]	Single-arm, pilot study	19 patients with distal lateral onychomycosis confirmed by culture	3 weekly NTAP treatments, performed monthly for 5 months	None	Safety (assessed by number of adverse events and subject-reported symptoms); clinical efficacy and mycological cure at month 6 follow-up	All but one patient met safety endpoints; 53.8% of patients achieved clinical cure while 15.4% achieved mycologic cure	Singeing of the nail due to faulty electrode with no long-term sequelae in one patient
Ahn et al.[43]	Single-arm, pilot study	5 patients with toenail onychomycosis	Single treatment of NTAP with three passes	None	Total number of fungal spores and fungal spore dispersion on reflectance confocal microscopy post-treatment	Immediately post-treatment, fungal spores became more disperse ($p = 0.5$); total number of spores decreased from 216 to 138 ($p = 0.31$)	Minor heating sensation

The near-infrared diode laser was studied for onychomycosis treatment. The device uses only 870- and 930-nm near-infrared light, wavelengths that are thought to have photolethal effects on fungal pathogens [33]. In a randomized controlled study of 26 patients with mild, moderate and severe onychomycosis of the toenails, patients received diode laser therapy treatment for a total of four sessions over 4 months. At day 180, 85% of treated toenails showed improvement with clear nail growth ($p=0.0015$). Overall, 65% of nails showed at least 3 mm and 26% showed at least 4 mm of clear nail growth, and 30% of nails had negative culture and periodic acid-Schiff [33].

Photodynamic therapy (PDT) has been investigated for onychomycosis treatment. PDT uses a light source to activate a photosensitizing agent applied topically or systemically and generates reactive oxygen species. Target fungi cells preferentially absorb the photosensitizer leading to destruction of cells by necrosis or apoptosis [34]. Photosensitizers fall into three categories: porphyrins, chlorophylls and dyes. Studies evaluating PDT for onychomycosis treatment have shown mixed results.

In a systematic review of 34 studies involving PDT treatment of onychomycosis ($n=380$ patients), treatment with methylene blue photosensitizer showed better complete cure rates (70%–80%) compared to 5-aminolevulinic acid-PDT (mycological cure rate 17%–57%) and methyl aminolevulinate-PDT (mycological cure rate 32%) (p value not reported) [35]. A more recent meta-analysis involving 18 studies and 343 patients with superficial fungal infections treated with PDT found an overall mycological cure rate of 55% (95% CI: 0.46–0.65); mycological cure rate using methylene blue was 67% (95% CI: 0.55–0.79, $p=0.03$), compared to 34% using 5-aminolevulinic acid (95% CI: 0.21–0.47, $p=0.87$) and 56% using methyl aminolevulinate (95% CI: 0.33–0.78, $p=0.10$) [36]. In a randomized, controlled, multicentre clinical trial comparing the effects of urea 40% plus methyl aminolevulinate-PDT (MAL-PDT) with urea 40% plus red light placebo PDT (pPDT) in 40 patients with onychomycosis, complete response (onychomycosis severity index=0) was observed in four patients (18.18%) in the MAL-PDT group compared to one patient (5.56%) in the pPDT group. Microbiological cure was achieved by seven patients (31.82%) in the MAL-PDT group compared to two patients (11.11%) in the pPDT group; no significant differences were observed between the treatment groups [37]. In a different study of 22 patients with toenail onychomycosis treated with PDT with methylene blue biweekly for 6 months, clinical response (not defined) was significantly higher in patients with mild-to-moderate onychomycosis (100%, CI: 100%) compared to patients with severe onychomycosis (63.6%, CI: 35%–92%) (p values not reported) [38].

In a prospective randomized study comparing outcomes from fractional CO_2 laser and methylene blue photodynamic therapy, 51 patients with onychomycosis were assigned to receive six CO_2 laser treatments, photodynamic therapy or a combination of both, with a follow-up period of 6 months [39]. Mean increase of proximal nail diameter (signifying clear nail) after treatment was highest in the combination group (52.94 ± 20.24), followed by the CO_2 group (43.82 ± 21.03) and the photodynamic therapy group (35.29 ± 17.0) ($p=0.044$) [39]. PDT may be a treatment option in onychomycosis patients who have failed other therapies or cannot continue other treatment due to adverse effects, although larger studies are warranted to better evaluate efficacy.

Non-thermal atmospheric plasma (NTAP) treatment has been studied for onychomycosis treatment. The mechanism of NTAP uses a dielectric insulator to create short pulses of strong electric field (approximately 20 kV/mm peak) that ionizes air molecules to create active chemical species such as ions, electrons, nitric oxide, ozone and hydroxyl radicals [40]. NTAP technologies have broad-spectrum antimicrobial effects that can be used to disinfect biotic and abiotic surfaces [41].

An initial study showed that NTAP inhibits *in vitro* growth of *T. rubrum* [42]. Several pilot studies using NTAP for the treatment of onychomycosis were subsequently conducted. In a pilot study evaluating NTAP in 19 patients with toenail onychomycosis, clinical cure was 53.8% while mycological cure was 15.4% (*p* value not reported). The majority of patients met the primary endpoint of safety and found the treatment was relatively painless [40]. In another pilot study assessing NTAP treatment in five patients with toenail onychomycosis, fungal cell wall disruption and hyphae breakage occurred following treatment, which decreased the number and dispersed clusters of spores [43]. Larger studies are needed to compare NTAP treatment alone with combination therapies.

9.5 Natural and Over-the-Counter Treatments

Given the need for more cost-effective options for patients with onychomycosis, there has been some study on the use of natural and over-the-counter (OTC) alternative treatments (Table 9.3). These non-traditional therapies may be less likely to promote antifungal resistance. Treatment options, including tea tree oil (TTO), essential oils (EO), natural coniferous resin (NCR) lacquer, ageratina pichinchensis (AP) and natural topical cough suppressants have shown antifungal activity in *in vitro* studies [44].

TTO, or melaleuca oil, is a near colourless, clear oil with broad-spectrum antimicrobial properties, and has been studied in a variety of dermatological conditions including acne and seborrhoeic dermatitis [45,46]. TTO has antifungal activity at a 5%–100% concentration, and is effective in treating tinea pedis [47]. A recent *in vitro* study assessing effectiveness of TTO against *T. rubrum* and *T. mentagrophytes* demonstrated growth inhibition at 0.04% and 0.07% oil concentrations, respectively ($p=0.004$, $p=0.017$) [48]. In a trial of 117 patients comparing 1% clotrimazole solution to 100% TTO, culture cure, confirmed by a negative culture test at 6 months, did not differ significantly between groups (11% vs. 18%, respectively; *p* value not reported) [49]. In another trial, 60 patients received treatment with 2% butenafine hydrochloride plus cream containing 5% TTO or a control cream containing TTO only three times daily for 8 weeks. Complete cure was higher in the active vs. placebo group (80% vs. 0%, $p<0.0001$) [50]. The combination treatment was effective for onychomycosis treatment; however, TTO alone showed no response [50]. In a prospective trial of 66 patients evaluating efficacy of 100% TTO applied twice daily for 6 months, 89% of patients achieved mycological cure and 27% of patients achieved clinical cure [46]. TTO has been well studied in both *in vitro* studies and clinical trials but was utilized in different formulations with some studies lacking control groups. Randomized controlled trials are needed to make evidence-based recommendations.

EOs may be good candidates for topical treatment of onychomycosis as they have low risk of fungal resistance and minimal side effects. EOs are composed of mixtures of natural substances from the distillation of aromatic plants, and are primarily composed of terpenes [51,52]. They have low molecular weight and therefore may penetrate the nail plate, allowing them to interact and interfere with fungal membranes and enzymatic reactions [51]. In a meta-analysis of 54 articles determining the efficacy of three common EOs (thyme, cinnamon, TTO) as therapy for onychomycosis against three fungal strains (*T. rubrum*, *T. mentagrophytes* and *Candida albicans*), the lowest MIC was observed with *Cinnamomum zeylanicum* EO (0.013–1120 µL/mL) against all three micro-organisms. The lowest minimum fungicidal concentration (MFC) was found for *Thymus vulgaris* EO (4.2 µL/mL) against

TABLE 9.3

Summary of Clinical Trial Results for Over the Counter Treatments

Study	Study Type	Study Participants	Intervention	Comparison	Primary Outcome Measures	Relevant Results	Relevant Adverse Effects
Tea Tree Oil							
Buck et al.[49]	Randomized, controlled, double-blind, multicentre trial	117 patients with distal onychomycosis confirmed by fungal culture	100% TTO topical treatment twice daily for 6 months	1% clotrimazole solution twice daily for 6 months	Culture cure at 6 months; clinical cure at 6 months	11% and 18% of patients in clotrimazole and TTO group, respectively, achieved culture cure; 61% and 60% of patient in clotrimazole and TTO group, respectively, achieved partial or complete clinical cure	Erythema and irritation in 7.8% of TTO patients
Syed et al.[50]	Randomized, placebo-controlled, double-blind trial	60 patients with onychomycosis confirmed by KOH and culture	Cream containing 5% TTO plus 2% butenafine hydrochloride applied three times daily under occlusion for 8 weeks	Cream containing 5% TTO only applied three times daily under occlusion for 8 weeks (20)	Mycological cure	80% and 0% of patients in the TTO + butenafine and TTO only group, respectively, achieved complete mycological cure ($p < 0.0001$)	Mild inflammation in 4% of TTO + butenafine patients
AbdelHamid et al.[46]	Randomized, double-blind, interventional cohort prospective trial	66 patients with onychomycosis confirmed by KOH and culture	100% TTO topical treatment twice daily for 6 months	None	Mycological cure at 6 months; clinical cure at 6 months	89% of patients achieved mycological cure; 27% of patients achieved complete clinical cure, 65% achieved partial clinical cure, 8% showed no clinical response ($p = 0.001$)	Dermatitis in 6% of patients

(Continued)

TABLE 9.3 *(Continued)*

Summary of Clinical Trial Results for Over the Counter Treatments

Study	Study Type	Study Participants	Intervention	Comparison	Primary Outcome Measures	Relevant Results	Relevant Adverse Effects
Natural Coniferous Resin							
Sipponen et al.[57]	Prospective, observational study	14 participants with clinical and mycological evidence of toenail onychomycosis	NCR topical treatment once daily for 9 months	None	Mycological cure	65% of patients achieved mycological cure (95% CI, 42%–87%)	None
Auvinen et al.[58]	Prospective, randomized, controlled, investigator-blinded trial	73 patients with onychomycosis confirmed by KOH and culture	Topical 30% NCR lacquer once daily for 9 months	Topical 5% amorolfine lacquer once weekly for 9 months or 250 mg oral terbinafine once daily for 3 months	Mycological cure at 10 months	13% (95% CI: 0–28), 8% (95% CI: 0–19) and 56% (95% CI: 35–77) of patients in the NCR, amorolfine and terbinafine groups, respectively, achieved complete mycological cure at 10 months ($p \le 0.002$)	None
Ageratina Pichinchensis							
Romero-Cerecero et al.[62]	Randomized, double-blind, controlled clinical trial	110 patients with mild-to-moderate onychomycosis confirmed by KOH	AP extract lacquer topical treatment for 6 months: every third day for first month, twice weekly for second month, weekly for 4 months	Ciclopirox 8% lacquer topical treatment for 6 months; every third day for first month, twice weekly for second month, weekly for 4 months	Mycological cure at 6 months	59.1% and 63.8% for the AP and ciclopirox groups, respectively, achieved mycological cure ($p = 0.328$)	None

(Continued)

TABLE 9.3 (*Continued*)

Summary of Clinical Trial Results for Over the Counter Treatments

Study	Study Type	Study Participants	Intervention	Comparison	Primary Outcome Measures	Relevant Results	Relevant Adverse Effects
Romero-Cerecero et al.[63]	Randomized, double-blind, controlled clinical trial	71 patients with mild-to-moderate onychomycosis and type II diabetes mellitus confirmed with culture	AP extract lacquer topical treatment for 6 months; once daily for 2 months, twice weekly for 4 months	Ciclopirox 8% lacquer topical treatment for 6 months; once daily for 2 months, twice weekly for 4 months	Mycological cure at 6 months; clinical cure at 6 months	7.1% and 8.6% of patients in the AP and ciclopirox groups, respectively, achieved mycological cure (no *p* value given); 71.4% and 68.6% of patients in the AP and ciclopirox groups, respectively, achieved partial clinical cure	Temporary skin irritation in skin surrounding the nail in 8.5% of AP patients
Romero-Cerecero et al.[64]	Randomized, double-blind, parallel clinical trial	122 patients with mild-to-moderate onychomycosis confirmed by culture	12.6% AP extract lacquer topical treatment for 6 months	16.8% AP extract lacquer topical treatment for 6 months	Clinical cure at 6 months	67.2% and 79.1% of patients in the 12.6% and 16.8% AP groups, respectively, achieved clinical cure (*p* = 0.01)	None
Ozonized Sunflower Oil							
Menendez et al.[65]	Randomized, simple-blinded, controlled clinical trial	400 patients with onychomycosis confirmed by culture	Ozonized sunflower oil (OLEOZON®) topical treatment twice daily for 3 months	Ketoconazole 2% cream twice daily for 3 months	Mycological and clinical cure at 3 months and 1 year	90.5% and 13.5% of patients in the ozonized sunflower oil and ketoconazole groups, respectively, achieved clinical and mycological cure at 3 months (*p* < 0.001); 2.8% and 37% of patients in the ozonized sunflower oil and ketoconazole groups, respectively, relapsed at 1 year	None

(*Continued*)

TABLE 9.3 (Continued)

Summary of Clinical Trial Results for Over the Counter Treatments

Vicks VapoRub

Study	Study Type	Study Participants	Intervention	Comparison	Primary Outcome Measures	Relevant Results	Relevant Adverse Effects
Derby et al.[66]	Clinical case-series, single-arm trial	18 patients with onychomycosis confirmed by culture	Vicks VapoRub topical treatment at least once daily for 48 weeks	None	Mycological and clinical cure at 48 weeks	27.8% of patients achieved mycological cure at 48 weeks; 22.2% of patients achieved complete clinical and mycological cure at 48 weeks; 55.6% of patients achieved partial clinical cure at 48 weeks	None
Snell et al.[67]	Single site, prospective pilot study	18 patients living with HIV infection with onychomycosis confirmed by dermatophyte test medium	Vicks VapoRub topical treatment at least once daily for 48 weeks	None	Clinical cure at 24 and 48 weeks	11% of patients achieved clinical cure and 83% of patients achieved partial clinical cure at 24 weeks; 53% of patients achieved partial clinical cure at 48 weeks	None

T. rubrum [53]. In a study comparing the antifungal activity of seven EOs incorporated into a green natural nail polish (GNNP) formulation against 10 dermatophyte strains, EOs showing greater inhibitory activity belonged to the genus of *Cymbopogon* (*C. giganteus*, *C. martini* and *C. citratus*), while EOs showing greater cytocidal activity were *C. martini* and *C. citratus* [52]. More studies are needed to further evaluate different EOs and their ability to treat onychomycosis.

NCR, derived from Norway spruce (*Picea abies*), has shown broad-spectrum antimicrobial activity against gram-positive bacteria and fungi in previous studies and is being explored as a topical treatment for onychomycosis [44,54–56]. In an observational study of 14 patients who applied NCR once daily for 9 months, 65% had mycological cure (95% CI, 42%–87%) [57]. In a different trial, 73 patients were assigned to received topical 30% NCR lacquer once daily for 9 months, topical 5% amorolfine lacquer once-weekly for 9 months or oral terbinafine 250 mg once daily for 3 months. Complete mycological cure rates at 10 months were 13%, 8% and 56%, respectively ($p \leq 0.002$) [58]. While oral terbinafine remains the gold standard of treatment, NCR showed similar antifungal efficacy to amorolfine with no adverse effects [58]. Larger randomized, controlled clinical trials are needed to make formal recommendations regarding NCR.

AP, historically used in Mexico for the treatment of fungal infections, has been investigated as a topical treatment for onychomycosis. AP extract has demonstrated *in vitro* antifungal activity in previous studies and has shown efficacy against tinea pedis in clinical trials [54,59–61]. In a clinical trial, 110 patients with onychomycosis received treatment with an AP extract lacquer or ciclopirox 8% lacquer for 6 months. Mycological cure rates were 59.1% and 63.8% for the AP and ciclopirox groups, respectively ($p=0.328$) [62]. A similar study comparing topical use of AP extract and ciclopirox in 71 patients with diabetes mellitus and onychomycosis showed mycological cure rates of 7.1% vs. 8.6%, respectively (p value not reported) [63]. Although the treatment of onychomycosis in diabetic patients may be more challenging, AP extract consistently showed similar efficacy to ciclopirox lacquer. A follow-up study comparing concentrations of 12.6% and 16.8% AP extract found the higher concentration significantly more effective at achieving clinical cure for onychomycosis ($p=0.01$), although larger trials are needed to make formal recommendations [64].

Ozonized sunflower oil, made by reacting ozone (O_3) with sunflower plant (*Helianthus annuus*) oil, demonstrated antifungal properties and has been used for treatment of tinea pedis [45]. A clinical trial of 400 patients evaluating efficacy for onychomycosis treatment, patients receiving treatment with topical ozonized sunflower oil (OLEOZON®), achieved greater mycological cure rates compared to patients using ketoconazole cream 2% (90.5% vs. 13.5%, $p<0.001$) [65].

Vicks VapoRub, an OTC topical cough suppressant, has been explored for onychomycosis treatment. It contains the ingredients camphor, eucalyptus oil and menthol that have previously demonstrated *in vitro* antifungal activity [45]. Two small clinical trials evaluating the efficacy of Vicks VapoRub applied daily for 48 weeks showed promising results, with the majority of patients showing substantial nail clearance and 5/18 (27.8%) patients achieving mycological cure [66,67]. However, all five patients had cultures positive for either *Candida parapsilosis* or *T. mentagrophytes*, and none of the other 13 patients with other organism growth achieved mycological cure ($p<0.001$). As these studies focus more on subjective measures of clinical appearance, larger clinical trials are needed to assess efficacy.

9.6 Conclusion

Effective treatment of onychomycosis is challenging for several reasons. The nail plate poses a barrier to antifungal drug penetration, and prolonged treatment periods are required due to slow nail growth and persistent fungal spores, which may contribute to patient non-compliance. The emergence of fungal resistance to existing treatments further diminishes their effectiveness, and the diverse range of fungal species causing onychomycosis adds complexity to treatment decisions. Patient-specific factors including comorbidities and preferences may influence available treatment options and outcomes, and many current systemic therapies have potential side effects and risk of drug interactions.

These challenges have spurred the exploration of emerging antifungal treatments and focus on novel approaches to address onychomycosis. Novel oral medications exhibit promising efficacy and safety profiles, showing potential superiority over current approved treatments, although more extensive research through larger clinical trials is warranted to comprehensively establish their comparative benefits. New and reformulated topical agents aim to enhance nail penetration, improve drug delivery and increase antifungal activity, often incorporating technologies to optimize drug release and penetration. Laser treatments and other device-based interventions are under investigation for onychomycosis management, but their efficacy remains to be conclusively established, necessitating more rigorous research and improved clinical outcomes. OTC and natural treatment options have also gained traction, offering accessible interventions for patients who may have limited therapy options. Development of these novel antifungal therapies is a balance between efficacy, safety and patient convenience, signalling a promising era in onychomycosis treatment.

References

1. Falotico JM, Lipner SR. Updated perspectives on the diagnosis and management of onychomycosis. *Clin Cosmet Investig Dermatol.* 2022;15:1933–57.
2. Krishna G, Ma L, Martinho M, Prasad P, et al. Determination of posaconazole levels in toenails of adults with onychomycosis following oral treatment with four regimens of posaconazole for 12 or 24 weeks. *Antimicrob Agents Chemother.* 2011;55(9):4424–6.
3. Elewski B, Pollak R, Ashton S, et al. A randomized, placebo- and active-controlled, parallel-group, multicentre, investigator-blinded study of four treatment regimens of posaconazole in adults with toenail onychomycosis. *Br J Dermatol.* 2012;166(2):389–98.
4. Gupta AK, Talukder M, Venkataraman M. Review of the alternative therapies for onychomycosis and superficial fungal infections: posaconazole, fosravuconazole, voriconazole, oteseconazole. *Int J Dermatol.* 2022;61(12):1431–41.
5. Sigurgeirsson B, van Rossem K, Malahias S, et al. A phase II, randomized, double-blind, placebo-controlled, parallel group, dose-ranging study to investigate the efficacy and safety of 4 dose regimens of oral albaconazole in patients with distal subungual onychomycosis. *J Am Acad Dermatol.* 2013;69(3):416–25.
6. Nakano M, Aoki Y, Yamaguchi H. Drug properties of fosravuconazole L-lysine ethanolate (NAILIN® Capsules 100mg), a new oral azole therapeutic for onychomycosis: an analysis based on non-clinical and clinical trial data. *Nihon Yakurigaku Zasshi.* 2019;153(2):79–87.

7. Watanabe S, Tsubouchi I, Okubo A. Efficacy and safety of fosravuconazole L-lysine ethanolate, a novel oral triazole antifungal agent, for the treatment of onychomycosis: a multicenter, double-blind, randomized phase III study. *J Dermatol*. 2018;45(10):1151–9.
8. Fávero MLD, Bonetti AF, Domingos EL, et al. Oral antifungal therapies for toenail onychomycosis: a systematic review with network meta-analysis toenail mycosis: network meta-analysis. *J Dermatolog Treat*. 2022;33(1):121–30.
9. Lipner SR. Pharmacotherapy for onychomycosis: new and emerging treatments. *Expert Opin Pharmacother*. 2019;20(6):725–35.
10. Elewski B, Brand S, Degenhardt T, et al. A phase II, randomized, double-blind, placebo-controlled, dose-ranging study to evaluate the efficacy and safety of VT-1161 oral tablets in the treatment of patients with distal and lateral subungual onychomycosis of the toenail. *Br J Dermatol*. 2021;184(2):270–80.
11. Gupta AK, Surprenant MS, Kempers SE, et al. Efficacy and safety of topical terbinafine 10% solution (MOB-015) in the treatment of mild to moderate distal subungual onychomycosis: a randomized, multicenter, double-blind, vehicle-controlled phase 3 study. *J Am Acad Dermatol*. 2021;85(1):95–104.
12. Blume-Peytavi U, Tosti A, Falqués M, et al. A multicentre, randomised, parallel-group, double-blind, vehicle-controlled and open-label, active-controlled study (versus amorolfine 5%), to evaluate the efficacy and safety of terbinafine 10% nail lacquer in the treatment of onychomycosis. *Mycoses*. 2022;65(4):392–401.
13. Ghannoum M, Isham N, Herbert J, et al. Activity of TDT 067 (terbinafine in Transfersome) against agents of onychomycosis, as determined by minimum inhibitory and fungicidal concentrations. *J Clin Microbiol*. 2011;49(5):1716–20.
14. Kawa N, Lee KC, Anderson RR, et al. Onychomycosis: a review of new and emerging topical and device-based treatments. *J Clin Aesthet Dermatol*. 2019;12(10):29–34.
15. Ullah KH, Rasheed F, Naz I, et al. Chitosan nanoparticles loaded poloxamer 407 Gel for transungual delivery of terbinafine HCl. *Pharmaceutics*. 2022;14(11):2353.
16. Baran R, Mailland F, Friscenda L, Caserini M. An innovative terbinafine transungual solution (P-3058): a phase 2b dose finding study in patients with mild to moderate onychomycosis. *J. Am. Acad. Dermatol*. 2014;70:AB88.
17. Del Rosso JQ. The role of topical antifungal therapy for onychomycosis and the emergence of newer agents. *J Clin Aesthet Dermatol*. 2014;7(7):10–8.
18. Iorizzo M, Hartmane I, Derveniece A, et al. Ciclopirox 8% HPCH nail lacquer in the treatment of mild-to-moderate onychomycosis: a randomized, double-blind amorolfine controlled study using a blinded evaluator [published correction appears in *Skin Appendage Disord*. 2016 May;1(4):168]. *Skin Appendage Disord*. 2016;1(3):134–40.
19. Baran R, Tosti A, Hartmane I, et al. An innovative water-soluble biopolymer improves efficacy of ciclopirox nail lacquer in the management of onychomycosis. *J Eur Acad Dermatol Venereol*. 2009;23(7):773–81.
20. Zalacain-Vicuña AJ, Nieto C, Picas J, et al. Efficacy and safety of a new medicated nail hydrolacquer in the treatment of adults with toenail onychomycosis: a randomised clinical trial *Mycoses*. 2023;66(7):566–575. doi: 10.1111/myc.13543.
21. Scher RK, Nakamura N, Tavakkol A. Luliconazole: a review of a new antifungal agent for the topical treatment of onychomycosis. *Mycoses*. 2014;57(7):389–93.
22. Watanabe S, Kishida H, Okubo A. Efficacy and safety of luliconazole 5% nail solution for the treatment of onychomycosis: a multicenter, double-blind, randomized phase III study. *J Dermatol*. 2017;44(7):753–9.
23. Takahata S, Kubota N, Takei-Masuda N, et al. Mechanism of action of ME1111, a novel antifungal agent for topical treatment of onychomycosis. *Antimicrob Agents Chemother*. 2015;60(2):873–80.
24. Kubota-Ishida N, Takei-Masuda N, Kaneda K, et al. *In Vitro* human onychopharmacokinetic and pharmacodynamic analyses of ME1111, a new topical agent for onychomycosis. *Antimicrob Agents Chemother*. 2017;62(1):e00779-17.

25. Hui X, Jung EC, Zhu H, et al. Antifungal ME1111 in vitro human onychopharmacokinetics. *Drug Dev Ind Pharm.* 2017;43(1):22–29.
26. Tabata Y, Takei-Masuda N, Kubota N, et al. Characterization of antifungal activity and nail penetration of ME1111, a new antifungal agent for topical treatment of onychomycosis. *Antimicrob Agents Chemother.* 2015;60(2):1035–9.
27. Gregoriou S, Kyriazopoulou M, Tsiogka A, et al. Novel and investigational treatments for onychomycosis. *J Fungi (Basel).* 2022;8(10):1079.
28. Mercer DK, Stewart CS, Miller L, et al. Improved methods for assessing therapeutic potential of antifungal agents against dermatophytes and their application in the development of NP213, a novel onychomycosis therapy candidate. *Antimicrob Agents Chemother.* 2019;63(5):e02117–18.
29. Mercer DK, Robertson JC, Miller L, et al. NP213 (Novexatin(r)): a unique therapy candidate for onychomycosis with a differentiated safety and efficacy profile. *Med Mycol.* 2020;58(8):1064–72.
30. Gupta AK, Paquet M. A retrospective chart review of the clinical efficacy of Nd:YAG 1064-nm laser for toenail onychomycosis. *J Dermatolog Treat.* 2015;26(4):376–8.
31. Ma W, Si C, Kasyanju Carrero LM, et al. Laser treatment for onychomycosis: a systematic review and meta-analysis. *Medicine (Baltimore).* 2019;98(48):e17948.
32. Gupta AK, Versteeg SG. A critical review of improvement rates for laser therapy used to treat toenail onychomycosis. *J Eur Acad Dermatol Venereol.* 2017;31(7):1111–18.
33. Landsman AS, Robbins AH, Angelini PF, et al. Treatment of mild, moderate, and severe onychomycosis using 870- and 930-nm light exposure. *J Am Podiatr Med Assoc.* 2010;100(3):166–77.
34. Bhatta AK, Keyal U, Wang XL. Photodynamic therapy for onychomycosis: a systematic review. *Photodiagnosis Photodyn Ther.* 2016;15:228–35.
35. Shen JJ, Jemec GBE, Arendrup MC, et al. Photodynamic therapy treatment of superficial fungal infections: a systematic review. *Photodiagnosis Photodyn Ther.* 2020;31:101774.
36. Dong Q, Kang Y, Zhang R. Treatment of superficial mycoses using photodynamic therapy: a systematic review and meta-analysis. *Photobiomodul Photomed Laser Surg.* 2023;41(2):37–47.
37. Gilaberte Y, Robres MP, Frías MP, et al. Methyl aminolevulinate photodynamic therapy for onychomycosis: a multicentre, randomized, controlled clinical trial. *J Eur Acad Dermatol Venereol.* 2017;31(2):347–54.
38. Souza LW, Souza SV, Botelho AC. Distal and lateral toenail onychomycosis caused by *Trichophyton rubrum*: treatment with photodynamic therapy based on methylene blue dye. *An Bras Dermatol.* 2014;89(1):184–6.
39. Sobhy N, Talla Eweed H, Omar SS. Fractional CO_2 laser-assisted methylene blue photodynamic therapy is a potential alternative therapy for onychomycosis in the era of antifungal resistance. *Photodiagnosis Photodyn Ther.* 2022;40:103149.
40. Lipner S, Friedman G, Scher R. Pilot study to evaluate a plasma device for the treatment of onychomycosis. *Clin Exp Dermatol.* 2017;42 (3):295–8.
41. Bulson JM, Liveris D, Derkatch I, et al. Non-thermal atmospheric plasma treatment of onychomycosis in an in vitro human nail model. *Mycoses.* 2020;63(2):225–32.
42. Heinlin J, Maisch T, Zimmermann JL et al. Contact-free inactivation of *Trichophyton rubrum* and *Microsporum canis* by cold atmospheric plasma treatment. *Future Microbiol* 2013; 8: 1097–106.
43. Ahn HJ, Kim TE, Lee YJ, et al. A pilot study of semiquantitative treatment evaluation following nonthermal atmospheric-pressure plasma administration for onychomycosis. *Skin Res Technol.* 2023;29(1):e13263.
44. Halteh P, Scher RK, Lipner SR. Over-the-counter and natural remedies for onychomycosis: do they really work? *Cutis.* 2016;98(5):E16–25.
45. Nickles MA, Lio PA, Mervak JE. Complementary and alternative therapies for onychomycosis: a systematic review of the clinical evidence. *Skin Appendage Disord.* 2022;8(4):269–79.
46. AbdelHamid D, Gomaa AHA, Mohammed GF, et al. Evaluation of the therapeutic efficacy of tea tree oil in treatment of onychomycosis. *Int J Pharmacogn Phytochem Res.* 2017;9(12):1414–20.
47. Satchell AC, Saurajen A, Bell C, et al. Treatment of interdigital tinea pedis with 25% and 50% tea tree oil solution: a randomized, placebo-controlled, blinded study. *Australas J Dermatol.* 2002;43(3):175–8.

48. Marcos-Tejedor F, González-García P, Mayordomo R. Solubilization in vitro of tea tree oil and first results of antifungal effect in onychomycosis. *Enferm Infecc Microbiol Clin* (Engl Ed). 2021;39(8):395–8.
49. Buck DS, Nidorf DM, Addino JG. Comparison of two topical preparations for the treatment of onychomycosis: *Melaleuca alternifolia* (tea tree) oil and clotrimazole. *J Fam Pract*. 1994;38(6):601–5.
50. Syed TA, Qureshi ZA, Ali SM, et al. Treatment of toenail onychomycosis with 2% butenafine and 5% *Melaleuca alternifolia* (tea tree) oil in cream. *Trop Med Int Health*. 1999;4(4):284–7.
51. Flores FC, Beck RC, da Silva C de B. Essential oils for treatment for onychomycosis: a mini-review. *Mycopathologia*. 2016;181(1–2):9–15.
52. Di Vito M, Scafuro C, Mariotti M, et al. Green natural nail polish modified with essential oils to treat onychomycosis. *Mycoses*. 2022;65(12):1127–36.
53. Villar Rodríguez J, Pérez-Pico AM, Mingorance-Álvarez E, et al. Meta-analysis of the anti-fungal activities of three essential oils as alternative therapies in dermatophytosis infections. *J Appl Microbiol*. 2022;133(2):241–53.
54. Rautio M, Sipponen A, Peltola R, et al. Antibacterial effects of home-made resin salve from Norway spruce (*Picea abies*). *APMIS*. 2007;115(4):335–40.
55. Rautio M, Sipponen A, Lohi J, et al. In vitro fungistatic effects of natural coniferous resin from Norway spruce (*Picea abies*). *Eur J Clin Microbiol Infect Dis*. 2012;31(8):1783–9.
56. Sipponen A, Peltola R, Jokinen JJ, et al. Effects of Norway spruce (*Picea abies*) resin on cell wall and cell membrane of *Staphylococcus aureus*. *Ultrastruct Pathol*. 2009;33(3):128–35.
57. Sipponen P, Sipponen A, Lohi J, et al. Natural coniferous resin lacquer in treatment of toenail onychomycosis: an observational study. *Mycoses*. 2013;56(3):289–96.
58. Auvinen T, Tiihonen R, Soini M, et al. Efficacy of topical resin lacquer, amorolfine and oral terbinafine for treating toenail onychomycosis: a prospective, randomized, controlled, investi-gator-blinded, parallel-group clinical trial. *Br J Dermatol*. 2015;173(4):940–8.
59. Navarro García VM, Gonzalez A, Fuentes M, et al. Antifungal activities of nine traditional Mexican medicinal plants. *J Ethnopharmacol*. 2003;87(1):85–8.
60. Sánchez-Ramos M, Marquina-Bahena S, Alvarez L, et al. Phytochemical, pharmacological, and biotechnological study of *Ageratina pichinchensis*: a native species of Mexico. *Plants (Basel)*. 2021;10(10):2225.
61. Romero-Cerecero O, Rojas G, Navarro V, et al. Effectiveness and tolerability of a standardized extract from *Ageratina pichinchensis* on patients with tinea pedis: an explorative pilot study controlled with ketoconazole. *Planta Med*. 2006;72(14):1257–61.
62. Romero-Cerecero O, Zamilpa A, Jiménez-Ferrer JE, et al. Double-blind clinical trial for evaluat-ing the effectiveness and tolerability of *Ageratina pichinchensis* extract on patients with mild to moderate onychomycosis. A comparative study with ciclopirox [published correction appears in *Planta Med*. 2008 Nov;74(14):1767]. *Planta Med*. 2008;74(12):1430–5.
63. Romero-Cerecero O, Islas-Garduño AL, Zamilpa A, et al. Effectiveness of an encecalin stan-dardized extract of *Ageratina pichinchensis* on the treatment of onychomycosis in patients with diabetes mellitus. *Phytother Res*. 2020;34(7):1678–86.
64. Romero-Cerecero O, Román-Ramos R, Zamilpa A, et al. Clinical trial to compare the effec-tiveness of two concentrations of the *Ageratina pichinchensis* extract in the topical treatment of onychomycosis. *J Ethnopharmacol*. 2009;126(1):74–8.
65. Menéndez S, Falcón L, Maqueira Y. Therapeutic efficacy of topical OLEOZON(r) in patients suffering from onychomycosis. *Mycoses*. 2011;54(5):e272–7.
66. Derby R, Rohal P, Jackson C, et al. Novel treatment of onychomycosis using over-the-counter mentholated ointment: a clinical case series. *J Am Board Fam Med*. 2011;24(1):69–74.
67. Snell M, Klebert M, Önen NF, et al. A novel treatment for onychomycosis in people liv-ing with HIV infection: Vicks VapoRub(tm) is effective and safe. *J Assoc Nurses AIDS Care*. 2016;27(1):109–13.

10

Preventive Measures

Eckart Haneke

Onychomycoses are often seen as the most common nail diseases. As with virtually all other diseases, prevention is better and easier than treatment. Prevention is often classified as primary to quaternary (Table 10.1).

Primary prevention of onychomycoses includes all measures to prevent a fungal infection that can spread to the nail apparatus. This includes avoiding the contact of fungal infection through fomites like contaminated nail care instruments, socks and shoes [1,2] but also of extension of a tinea of the surrounding skin to the nail [3]. Further, the role of public swimming pools, sports facilities, mats in dojos, etc., is important. As it is virtually impossible to keep these facilities fungus-free the use of antifungal preparations for the feet after their use is often stressed. It must be kept in mind that by far the most common route of infection is via the hyponychium, and careful examination of the skin of hands and feet very often reveals some fine squames that, upon mycologic investigation, prove to be infected by fungi. Thus, consistent therapy of tinea manuum et pedum is an important preventive measure.

Hands and feet should be kept dry and clean and washed with soap, particularly after sweating and swimming as fungal spores need some humidity to stick to the stratum corneum and grow out infective hyphae. The nails of all digits should be kept short and clean to avoid moisture under them that would favour fungal growth as moist keratin

TABLE 10.1

Levels of Prevention for Onychomycoses

Level	Definition
Primary prevention	Methods to avoid occurrence of onychomycosis either by eliminating pathogenic fungi or increasing resistance to infection. Examples include treatment of potential predisposing factors, household and personal hygienic measures, and avoiding smoking.
Secondary prevention	Methods to detect and address an existing mycosis of the skin surrounding the nails or already existing onychomycosis prior to the appearance of symptoms.
Tertiary prevention	Methods to reduce the signs and damage of symptomatic disease, such as nail destruction, adverse drug reactions, severe foot infections such as erysipelas, worsening of diabetic foot, reduction of quality of life and decrease of self-esteem. Examples also include procedures that halt the spread or progression of infection.
Quaternary prevention	Methods to mitigate or avoid results of unnecessary or excessive interventions in the health system, including the sequelae of serious adverse drug reactions, particularly in case of incorrect diagnosis, e.g. AGNUS treated as onychomycosis and then serious adverse drug effects, as well as potential violations of rights.

Source: Adapted for Onychomycosis and modified from https://en.wikipedia.org/wiki/Preventive_health-care, last accessed 6 Sept 2023.

DOI: 10.1201/9781003381648-11

is the favourite feeding substance for keratinophilic fungi such as dermatophytes. The wearing of open shoes such as sandals also allows the feet to stay dry. Flip-flops in public swimming pools, sports halls, locker rooms and communal saunas prevents direct contact of the feet with potentially fungus-containing keratin squames on the floor. Nail clippers, scissors, files and other nail grooming instruments should not be shared with others. Effective exhaustion of nail dust in nail parlours is mandatory [4]. People with athlete's foot should treat their interdigital mycosis right away to prevent the spread of this mycotic infection to the surrounding sole of the foot and to the tip of the toes from where the infection may spread under the hyponychium and into the nail bed. Breathable socks made from natural materials such as cotton or wool permit evaporation of moisture and keep the feet dry. Socks should be changed every day and preferably also shoes in order to let them thoroughly dry. Shoes may be disinfected using antifungal powder or sprays. In older times, the shoes were thoroughly "sterilized" by inserting a formalin-soaked cotton ball into the tip of the shoe, putting the shoe into a plastic bag, closing it air-tight and leaving it for 24 hours in a warm corner; the cotton ball was then removed, and the shoes ventilated for at least 48 hours. This is no longer done although this was probably the most efficient way to kill all potential pathogens; the smell of formaldehyde is very unpleasant and the procedure is often felt to be too tedious; however, sufficient ventilation reduced the risk of formaldehyde allergy virtually to nil.

Most dermatophytes are zoonotic, and close contact with pets generates an increased risk of infection. Dermatophytoses are most frequent where animals are in the household, and their incidence increases with the growing popularity of pets worldwide [5]. Poor hygiene as experienced by the homeless is also a risk factor [6].

As the susceptibility to get onychomycosis appears to be an autosomal dominant trait – as seen very often by the vertical spread of onychomycosis in the family – no-one should go barefoot in the household, particularly in the bathroom, but always wear slippers or flip-flops. The floor should be wiped wet at least once a week with addition of a mild disinfective agent. All family members should consult a dermatologist if someone has signs of a tinea or onychomycosis.

It is thought that nail polish can harden the nail and create a barrier impeding fungal penetration into the nail. Immunocompromised persons should be particularly aware of their heightened risk to acquire a fungal infection.

Secondary prevention includes all methods to detect and address an existing onychomycosis before the development of symptoms, particularly the early treatment of single mycotic nails before the disease spreads to more nails. Early targeted treatment after confirmation of the onychomycosis and exclusion of any nail condition looking clinically similar to an onychomycosis is mandatory. The asymmetric gait nail unit syndrome (AGNUS) is an extremely common condition and closely mimics onychomycosis [7]. Classically, it is not associated with fungal infection, but environmental fungi may colonize such a nail [8].

Onychomycosis treatment is often not satisfying as even long-term treatment with a highly effective antifungal drug may remain unsuccessful; this is proof of the fact that there might be more factors to be considered when treating a patient with onychomycosis [9]. The genetic background has already been mentioned. The importance of previous trauma for the development of fungal nail infections has long been known; however, single-digit onychomycosis may be extremely recalcitrant, and a careful patient history is necessary to find out a previous trauma to this specific digit [10]. Despite an excellent therapeutic response to terbinafine (82% clinical cure or with minimal residual lesions as well as 82% mycological cure maintained after 2 years), long-term results for some patients with onychomycosis treated with systemic antifungals are somewhat disappointing [11–13].

A study reported the 3-year follow-up of a group of 47 "cured" patients with toenail ony-chomycosis using a 4-month course of either terbinafine or itraconazole. The relapses were more common in patients treated with pulsed itraconazole (36.3%) than in patients treated with continuous (16.6%) or intermittent (15.3%) terbinafine. This was confirmed in a double-blind comparative trial of terbinafine 250 mg/day versus itraconazole 200 mg/day for 12 weeks [9,14]. In another study of 88 patients, 36 weeks after cessation of 12 weeks of itraconazole (continuous or pulse) therapy, total clinical cure was achieved in 35% of these patients, 93% of whom had negative cultures. At a follow-up at week 104, the total clinical cure was 39%, with negative cultures in 57%. Younger patients showed significantly better clinical cure rates at week 36 than older patients, possibly due to faster nail growth [15]. While the latter studies have indicated that in some cases there are low long-term remission rates with itraconazole, there have also been studies showing similar results for terbinafine. For instance, patients treated with 250 mg terbinafine daily for 3–6 months were followed for approximately 2.5 years. Although the status of some patients changed from "cured" to "not cured" and vice versa, nearly half of the patients were clinically cured after 1 year and had clinical and mycological cure at 2.5 years [16].

10.1 Reasons for Prevention

These studies suggest that the long-term chances for cure are unsatisfactory for some patients receiving treatment for fungal nail infections because of treatment failure, relapse and re-infection. A more recent and aggravating problem is the emergence of drug resistance, particularly in infections due to *Trichophyton indotineae* [17–19].

Failure of treatment of onychomycosis may be due to re-infection or – very often – to incomplete eradication of the original fungus by treatment (relapse) (see Table 10.2). However, in most cases it is virtually impossible to differentiate re-infections from true relapses. Failures that occur within 1 year after stop of treatment are more likely to be recurrences following recrudescence of the pre-existing infection, whereas failures that occur later may be re-infections (new infections). The latter should account for about two-thirds of relapses. So, why are patients with onychomycosis so easily re-infected? Susceptibility to onychomycosis depends on several factors, including genetic predisposition, reduced nail growth rate and a variety of underlying diseases, and most of these predisposing factors are either not considered in the treatment of the patient or not amenable to therapy.

10.1.1 Genetic Predisposition

A genetic predisposition to *Trichophyton* onychomycosis has already been reported in 1921 [20]. *Trichophyton rubrum* onychomycosis frequently occurs in several members of the same family in different generations. *T. rubrum* infection, however, is rare in persons marrying into infected families (if they do not come from a family that also has *T. rubrum* infection), suggesting a genetic predisposition rather than an intrafamilial transmission of the infection [21,22]. It is often associated with atopy, and the prevalence is also higher in those with psoriasis [23]. Pedigree studies suggest an autosomal dominant inheritance [24]. Predisposed individuals acquire *T. rubrum* infection in early childhood from their infected parents. The infection remains localized to the plantar region for many years without being noticed by the patient. Nail invasion, which usually begins in adult life, is possibly favoured by local factors such as reduced nail growth rate and trauma. Genetic predisposition to *T. rubrum* invasion may possibly be linked to biochemical abnormalities in the keratins. A genetic susceptibility to infection by *T. concentricum* (tinea imbricata) has also been found [25]. HLA-DR8 may be a susceptibility gene for onychomycosis [26], whereas HLA-DR4 might exert a certain protective role [27]. CARD9 (caspase recruitment domain–containing protein 9) deficiency due to compound heterozygous mutations [28], and responsible genes encoding interleukin-22, β-defensin 2 and 4 [29] as well as genetic defects in dectin-1, which increased the prevalence of the disease in families, are involved in the inheritance of the susceptibility in their members [30].

Gender has a role in determining the risk that an individual will develop onychomycosis [31]. In one survey, the odds of males having onychomycosis were 84.3% greater than females of the same age [32].

The presence of infectious fungi is not always associated with an onychomycosis [33], although short-term mechanical carriage of infectious dermatophytes on the skin and under the nail poses a risk for transmission. Chronic fungal carriers (months to years) as well as asymptomatic infections are a risk for all contact persons.

10.1.2 Reduced Nail Growth Rate

It has been suggested that onychomycosis affects the toenails of elderly individuals because of slow growth rate [34]. This is probably also the reason why toenail infections are about seven times more frequent than fingernail mycoses. The association between onychomycosis and ageing is very well established [35] and the prevalence of the disease is expected to increase in the coming decades due to the increasing longevity of the human population [36].

10.1.3 Underlying Diseases

10.1.3.1 Nail Diseases

Onycholysis and nail bed hyperkeratosis may favour nail invasion by fungi. This explains why onychomycosis is quite common in patients with traumatic nail dystrophies or nail bed psoriasis. Onychomycosis is more common in patients with psoriasis with a prevalence ranging from 13% to 21.5%. It has been shown that psoriasis increases by 50% the risk of developing onychomycosis [37].

10.1.3.2 Dermatological Diseases

Dermatophyte infection is often observed in patients with palmoplantar keratoderma or ichthyosis [38,39].

10.1.3.3 Orthopaedic Abnormalities

Close inspection of the feet in patients with toenail changes is essential and very often reveals slight to obvious foot deformation [40]. Foot and toe deformation increases the mechanical stress and strain to the toenail region resulting in onycholysis, subungual hyperkeratosis and growth abnormality, thus reducing the nail growth rate and both increasing the susceptibility to infection as well as decreasing the chances of successful antifungal therapy [41]. More than a quarter of professional dancers were found to have onychomycosis [42].

10.1.3.4 Systemic Disease

Peripheral vascular disorders and diabetes mellitus have frequently been reported to predispose to onychomycosis.

10.1.3.4.1 Diabetes Mellitus

Diabetes mellitus is the most prevalent metabolic disease around the world. Organ dysfunction, immunodeficiency, vascular complications and peripheral neuropathy are frequent sequelae contributing to susceptibility to fungal and bacterial infections of the nails [43]. The association between onychomycosis and diabetes has been confirmed by several studies and we can assume that diabetics are three times more susceptible to onychomycosis than non-diabetics [44,45]. Severe diabetes may lead to the diabetic foot with a very high risk of bacterial and fungal infections.

Immunosuppression clearly predisposes to onychomycosis. In temperate climate, nail invasion by *Candida* is almost exclusively seen in patients with impaired immune function.

Patients with HIV infection are more commonly affected by onychomycosis than healthy individuals [46]. Predisposing factors among HIV-positive patients include low CD4 count, familial history of onychomycosis, personal history of tinea pedis and walking barefoot around swimming pools [47].

Other diseases which have been associated with onychomycosis include Cushing's syndrome [48], peripheral neuropathies, lymphoma [49], atopic disorders, cancer, rheumatoid diseases and gastrointestinal disorders [50].

In some cases, nail infection may become the portal of entry for erysipelas or a disseminated infection. Proximal subungual onychomycosis due to *T. rubrum* is often observed in HIV patients, where it is considered to be a negative prognostic feature. For this reason, patients with *T. rubrum* proximal subungual onychomycosis should be examined for the presence of underlying immunosuppression.

10.1.3.5 Cigarette Smoking

Cigarette smoking has also been found to increase the risk of developing onychomycosis [51].

10.1.3.6 Post-therapeutic Prevention

Since relapses of onychomycosis are frequent, consideration should be given to prevention of recurrences in patients who have been cured. High rates of infections have been associated with working conditions where:

- Workers are required to wear heavy duty shoes or are exposed to wet conditions, which create a confined, damp and warm atmosphere that facilitates the development of fungal and bacterial infection.
- Industries which do not provide sufficient information to workers about the importance of foot hygiene.
- Jobs that necessitate the use of communal showers, which can lead to recurrent fungal contamination.

TABLE 10.2

Individuals at Risk

Armed forces, police
Athletes
Dustmen
Employees of indoor swimming pools
Excavation workers
Mine workers
Nuclear fuel workers
Rubber industry workers
Sewer workers
Steel and furnace workers
Wood-cutters

10.1.3.7 Collective Preventive Measures

These are generally ineffective because they are difficult to apply and/or not adhered to. *Ideally* the following situations are desirable [52]:

- Tiled shower floors should be inclined to allow sufficient drainage and non-stagnation of wastewater (*T. rubrum* survives for 25 days in stagnant water at 23°C–25°C).

- Wooden shower-floor grids should be replaced by plastic ones to limit the adhesion of scales shed by infected feet.

- Floors of communal showers must be washed and disinfected at least once daily with, for example, sodium hypochlorite, if possible after use by each group of workers.

Individual preventive measures have to be added to the collective preventive measures.

Although generally recommended, there is still no scientific proof that disinfecting shoes and socks, though logical, affects the course or relapse rate of onychomycosis. However, it is important to treat recurrent tinea pedis at the earliest opportunity. In individuals at risk for tinea pedis (Table 10.2), it is important to limit spread in shower rooms by providing disposable slippers and by careful foot hygiene including drying the web spaces after showering.

There are many antifungals and disinfective agents used prophylactically in tinea pedum and onychomycoses, such as tolnaftate [53], neticonazole [54], ciclopirox olamine and bifonazole powder [55], efinaconazole [56], to prevent recurrent tinea pedis. A weekly application of terbinafine cream in the nail area [57], between the toes and on the soles of the feet would also be expected to be effective in preventing re-infection in those individuals who appear to be particularly susceptible to onychomycosis. A once-weekly application of an antifungal nail varnish has also been recommended [58].

Finally, long-term intermittent therapy might prevent the re-establishment of tinea pedis and limit the risk of nail re-infection. Periodic use of transungual antifungal drug delivery systems, which are retained in nail keratin after discontinuation of therapy, appears to be a logical and safe method for preventing recurrences. However, it is doubtful if such approaches are practicable in the majority of patients and good foot hygiene at home or in the workplace coupled with early treatment of recurrent tinea pedis may provide the best solution.

10.2 Conclusion

Age, obesity, tinea pedis, peripheral vascular disease, venous insufficiency, diabetes mellitus and HIV are significant risk factors for onychomycosis; their treatment is necessary for effective prevention [59].

References

1. Gupta AK, Simkovich AJ, Hall DC. The march against onychomycosis: a systematic review of the sanitization methods for shoes, socks, and textiles. *J Am Podiatr Med Assoc.* 2022;112(4):21–223.
2. Skaastrup KN, Astvad KMT, Arendrup MC, et al. Disinfection trials with terbinafine-susceptible and terbinafine-resistant dermatophytes. *Mycoses.* 2022;65(7):741–6.
3. Albucker SJ, Falotico JM, Choo ZN, et al. Risk factors and treatment trends for onychomycosis: a case-control study of onychomycosis patients in the all of us research program. *J Fungi (Basel).* 2023;9(7):712–18.
4. Song W, Matthapan L, Bunyaratavej S, et al. Efficacy of a newly developed inward airflow safety cabinet to prevent the spread of infected nail dust particles during mechanical nail reduction in onychomycosis. *J Am Podiatr Med Assoc.* 2022;112(2):20–200.
5. Łagowski D, Gnat S, Nowakiewicz A, et al. The prevalence of symptomatic dermatophytoses in dogs and cats and the pathomechanism of dermatophyte infections. *Postępy Mikrobiol – Adv Microbiol.* 2019;58:165–76.
6. Rasul TF, Gamret AC, Morgan O, et al. Cutaneous fungal infections in patients experiencing homelessness and treatment in low-resource settings: a scoping review. *Cureus.* 2022;14(10):e30840.
7. Zaias N, Escovar SX, Rebell G. Opportunistic toenail onychomycosis. The fungal colonization of an available nail unit space by non-dermatophytes is produced by the trauma of the closed shoe by an asymmetric gait or other trauma. A plausible theory. *J Eur Acad Dermatol Venereol.* 2014;28(8):1002–6.
8. Zaias N, Escovar SX, Zaiac MN, et al. Onychomycosis, the active invasion of a normal nail unit by a dermatophytic versus the colonization of an existing abnormal nail unit by environmental fungus. *Skinmed.* 2020;18(1):18–22.
9. Scher RK, Baran R. Onychomycosis in clinical practice: factors contributing to recurrence. *Br J Dermatol.* 2003;149 S65:5–9.
10. Haneke E, Stovbyr G. Post-traumatic single-digit onychomycosis. *J Fungi (Basel).* 2023;9(3):313–19.
11. De Cuyper C. Long-term evaluation of terbinafine 250 and 500 mg daily in a 16-week oral treatment for toenail onychomycosis. *Br J Dermatol.* 1996;135:156–7.
12. Bräutigam M. Terbinafine versus itraconazole: a controlled clinical comparison in onychomycosis of the toenails. *J Am Acad Dermatol.* 1998;38:S53–6.
13. De Backer M, De Vroey C, Lesaffre E, et al. Twelve weeks of continuous oral therapy for toenail onychomycosis caused by dermatophytes: a double-blind comparative trial of terbinafine 250 mg/day, versus itraconazole 200 mg/day. *J Am Acad Dermatol.* 1998;38:S57–63.
14. Tosti A, Piraccini BM, Stinchi C, et al. Relapses of onychomycosis after successful treatment with systemic antifungals: a three-year follow-up. *Dermatology* 1998;197:162–6.
15. Heikkilä H, Stubb S. Long-term results of patients with onychomycosis treated with itraconazole. *Acta Derm Venereol.* 1997;77:70–1.
16. Brandrup F, Larsen PO. Long-term follow-up of toe-nail onychomycosis treated with terbinafine. *Acta Derm Venereol.* 1997;77:238.

17. Saunte DM, Hare RK, Jørgensen KM, et al. Emerging terbinafine resistance in trichophyton: clinical characteristics, squalene epoxidase gene mutations, and a reliable EUCAST method for detection. *Antimicrob Agents Chemother.* 2019;63:e01126-19.

18. Gupta AK, Renaud HJ, Quinlan EM, et al. The growing problem of antifungal resistance in onychomycosis and other superficial mycoses. *Am J Clin Dermatol.* 2021;22:149–57.

19. Hwang JK, Bakotic WL, Gold JAW, et al. Isolation of terbinafine-resistant *Trichophyton rubrum* from onychomycosis patients who failed treatment at an academic center in New York, United States. *J Fungi (Basel).* 2023;9(7):710.

20. Hodges RS. Ringworm of the nails: a preliminary report of sixteen cases of onychomycosis with a cultural study of twelve of these cases due to *Trichophytons. Arch Derm Syphilol.* 1921;4:1–26.

21. Gnat S, Łagowski D, Nowakiewicz A. Genetic predisposition and its heredity in the context of increased prevalence of dermatophytoses. *Mycopathologia* 2021;186(2):163–76.

22. García-Romero MT, Arenas R. New insights into genes, immunity, and the occurrence of dermatophytosis. *J Invest Dermatol.* 2015;135:655–7.

23. Hanifin JM, Ray LF, Lobitz Jr WC. Immunological reactivity in dermatophytosis. *Br J Dermatol.* 1974;90:1–8.

24. Zaias N, Tosti A, Rebell G, et al. Autosomal dominant pattern of distal subungual onychomycosis caused by *Trichophyton rubrum. J Am Acad Dermatol.* 1996;34:302–4.

25. Hay RJ, Reid S, Talwat E, et al. Endemic tinea imbricate–a study on Goodenough Island, Papua New Guinea. *Trans R Soc Trop Med Hyg.* 1984;78(2):246–51.

26. Carrillo-Meléndrez H, Ortega-Hernández E, Granados J, et al. Role of HLA-DR alleles to increase genetic susceptibility to onychomycosis in nail psoriasis. *Skin Appendage Disord.* 2016;2:22–5.

27. Zaitz C, Campbell I, Moraes JR, et al. HLA-associated susceptibility to chronic onychomycosis in Brazilian Ashkenazic Jews. *Int J Dermatol.* 1996;35:681–2.

28. Nazarian RM, Lilly E, Gavino C, et al. Novel CARD9 mutation in a patient with chronic invasive dermatophyte infection (tinea profunda) *J Cutan Pathol.* 2020;47:166–70.

29. Jaradat SW, Cubillos S, Krieg N, et al. Low DEFB4 copy number and high systemic hBD-2 and IL-22 levels are associated with dermatophytosis. *J Invest Dermatol.* 2015;135:750–8.

30. Ferwerda B, Ferwerda G, Plantinga TS, et al. Human dectin-1 deficiency and mucocutaneous fungal infections. *N Engl J Med.* 2009;361:1760–7.

31. Elewski BE, Charif MA. Prevalence of onychomycosis in patients attending a dermatology clinic in northeastern Ohio for other conditions. *Arch Dermatol.* 1997;133(9):1172–3.

32. Gupta AK, Jain HC, Lynd CW, et al. Prevalence and epidemiology of unsuspected onychomycosis in patients visiting dermatologists offices in Ontario, Canada. A multicenter survey of 2001 patients. *Int J Dermatol.* 1998;36:783–7.

33. Baran R, Badillet G. Primary onycholysis of the big toenails: a review of 113 cases. *Br J Dermatol.* 1982;106(5):529–34.

34. Orentreich N, Markofsky JV, Ogelman JH. The effect of aging on the rate of linear nail growth. *J Invest Dermatol.* 1979;73:126–30.

35. Haneke E, Roseeuw D. The scope of onychomycosis: epidemiology and clinical features. *Int J Dermatol.* 1999;38(Suppl 2):7–12.

36. Burzykowski T, Molenberghs G, Abeck D, et al. High prevalence of foot diseases in Europe: results of the Achilles project. *Mycoses* 2003;46:496–505.

37. Larsen GK, Haedersdal M, Sveigaard EL. The prevalence of onychomycosis in patients with psoriasis and other skin diseases. *Acta Derm Venereol.* 2003;83:206–20.

38. Nielsen PG, Faergemann J. Dermatophytes and keratin in patients with hereditary palmoplantar keratoderma. *Acta Derm Venereol.* 1993;73:416–18.

39. Hay RJ. Chronic dermatophyte infections. Clinical and mycological features. *Br J Dermatol.* 1982;106:1–7.

40. Murray SC, Dawber RP. Onychomycosis of toenails: orthopaedic and podiatric considerations. *Australas J Dermatol.* 2002;43(2):105–12.

41. Haneke E. Toenails: where orthopedics and onychology meet. In: Baran R, editor. *Advances in Nail Disease and Management*. Cham, Switzerland: Springer Nature; 2021. pp. 71–86.

42. Zahn R, Schmidt M, Wallner A, et al. Work-related dermatoses of the feet in professional dancers: a pilot study. *Med Probl Perform Art*. 2023;38(1):16–22.

43. Korpowska K, Majchrzycka M, Adamski Z. The assessment of prophylactic and therapeutic methods for nail infections in patients with diabetes. *Postepy Dermatol Alergol*. 2022;39(6):1048–52.

44. Gupta AK, Konnikov N, MacDonald P, et al. Prevalence and epidemiology of toenail onychomycosis in diabetic subject: a multicentre survey. *Br J Dermatol*. 1998;139:665–71.

45. Agrawal S, Singal A, Grover C, et al. Prevalence of onychomycosis in patients with diabetes mellitus: a cross-sectional study from a tertiary care hospital in North India. *Indian J Dermatol Venereol Leprol*. 2023;89(5):710–17.

46. Daniel CR III, Norton LA, Scher RK. The spectrum of nail disease in patients with human immunodeficiency virus infection. *J Am Acad Dermatol*. 1992;27:93–9.

47. Gupta AK, Taborda P, Taborda V, et al. Epidemiology and prevalence of onychomycosis in HIV-positive individuals. *In J Dermatol*. 2000;39:746–53.

48. Nelson LM, McNiece KJ. Recurrent Cushing's syndrome with *Trichophyton rubrum* infection. *Arch Dermatol*. 1959;80:700–4.

49. Lewis GM, Hopper ME, Scott MJ. Generalised *Trichophyton rubrum* infection associated with systemic lymphoblastoma. *Arch Derm*. 1953;67:247–62.

50. Sigurgeirsson B, Steingrimsson O. Risk factors associated with onychomycosis. *J Eur Acad Dermatol Venereol*. 2004;18:48–51.

51. Gupta AK, Gupta MA, Summerbell RC, et al. The epidemiology of onychomycosis: possible role of smoking and peripheral arterial disease. *J Eur Acad Dermatol Venereol*. 2000;14:466–9.

52. Baran R. Onychomycosis. In Grob JJ, Stern RS, MacKie RM, et al., editors. *Epidemiology, Causes and Prevention of Skin Diseases*. Oxford: Blackwell; 1997. pp. 276–8.

53. Smith EB, Dickson JE, Knox JM. Tolnafate powder in prophylaxis of tinea pedis. *South Med J*. 1974;67:776–8.

54. Albanese G, Cintio R, Giorgetti P, et al. Recurrent tinea pedis: a double blind study on the prophylactic use of fenticonazole powder. *Mycoses* 1992;35:157–9.

55. Galimberti RL, Belli L, Negroni R, et al. Prophylaxis of tinea pedis interdigitalis with bifonazole 1% powder. *Dermatologica* 1984;169(Suppl 1):111–16.

56. Lipner SR, Joseph WS, Vlahovic TC, et al. Therapeutic recommendations for the treatment of toenail onychomycosis in the US. *J Drugs Dermatol*. 2021;20(10):1076–84.

57. Evans EG, Seaman RA, James IG. Short-duration therapy with terbinafine 1% cream in dermatophyte skin infections. *Br J Dermatol*. 1994;130:83–7.

58. Zalacain-Vicuña AJ, Nieto C, Picas J, et al. Efficacy and safety of a new medicated nail hydrolacquer in the treatment of adults with toenail onychomycosis: a randomised clinical trial. *Mycoses* 2023;66(7):566–75.

59. Frazier WT, Santiago-Delgado ZM, Stupka KC 2nd. Onychomycosis: rapid evidence review. *Am Fam Physician* 2021;104(4):359–67.

Part 2

Hair

11

Epidemiology of Scalp Infection

Kelati Awatef

11.1 Introduction

Dermatophyte fungi are organisms specifically adapted to invade keratinized tissue such as the epidermis and the hair [1] (Figure 11.1). Tinea capitis (TC) or scalp ringworm is a highly contagious superficial fungal infection of the scalp and its associated hair follicles [2,3]. It is one of commonest infectious diseases in the paediatric population [4], as it accounts for 25%–30% of all fungal infections [5], especially in preadolescent children. Due to many factors, its epidemiological characteristics and pathogenic strain distribution in children vary not only all over the world but also may change over time even in the same region [6].

11.1.1 Transmission of Organisms

These organisms causing TC are classified as zoophilic, anthropophilic and geophilic dermatophytes depending on whether they are acquired through direct contact with infected animals, transmitted from one infected human to another, or contracted from contaminated soil or fomites such as hair care utensils or toys. The indirect way of transmission is assumed to be predominant as dermatophytes transmit primarily through the shedding of infected hairs and skin cells [7].

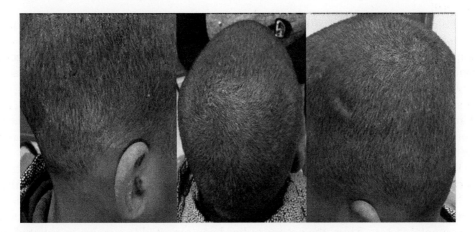

FIGURE 11.1
Trichophytic tinea capitis with diffuse scaling of the scalp (*Trichophyton violaceum*).

DOI: 10.1201/9781003381648-13

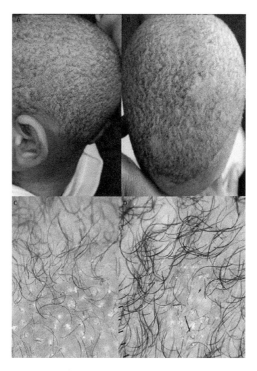

FIGURE 11.2
Microsporum audouinii tinea capitis in a 5-year-old boy from Gabon: (a,b) Sharply demarcated, round, alopecic patches with variable size and hair shafts breaking off close to the surface and discrete skin scaling better visualized using dermoscopy (c and d).

Anthropophilic dermatophytes such as *Tricophyton violaceum*, *Tricophyton tonsurans*, *Tricophyton schoenleinii*, *Tricophyton soudanense*, *Tricophyton rubrum* and *Microsporum audouinii* are usually responsible for endemic infections (Figure 11.2), while zoophilic dermatophytes such as *Microsporum canis*, *Trichophyton mentagrophytes* and *Trichophyton verrucosum*, and geophilic dermatophytes (*Microsporum gypseum*) are responsible for sporadic infections [2,8,9].

TC could also be asymptomatic when dermatophytes are detected on the scalp of persons without signs or symptoms of infection; these asymptomatic carriers are presumed to contribute to the transmission and persistence of the dermatophyte, and new infections in communities [7]. This is why detection and prophylactic treatment of close contacts to patients with anthropophilic dermatophytes is recommended in most guidelines [7,10]. Also, sources of zoophilic infections (*M. canis* for example) such as cats, dogs, horses, monkeys and rabbits may also be asymptomatic carriers, and harbour the pathogen in their fur without showing clinical signs [10,11]. This may prevent and counteract control measures in the community by maintaining the population of pathogens.

On the other hand, in the chronic inflammatory dermatophyte infection of the scalp or tinea capitis favosa, the organism (mainly anthropophilic *T. schoenleinii*) grows within the hair shaft (endothrix favosa), and this is why favus is less contagious than other dermatophytoses, and the pathogen is much less accessible for the host's immune defence and environmental factors. Thus, the organism has been reported to survive in epilated hairs for up to 54 months [12].

11.1.2 Epidemiology

TC has a high prevalence in the paediatric population all over the world. It is most common in hot, humid climates such as Africa, Southeast Asia and Central America [13]. It is also influenced by multiple factors, such as economic development, changes in lifestyle, immigration and animal distribution [14].

In the early 20th century, it was particularly linked to a considerable social stigma, because of its association with poverty and overpopulation [1,15].

After the discovery of griseofulvin by the 1960s, a simple therapeutic programme was performed in order to control this endemic problem in Europe and USA and other countries, to identify the infected cases, often at school, and to treat them by using single doses of griseofulvin administered through a supervised dosing schedule, which finally led to the elimination of scalp ringworm, most commonly caused by *M. audouinii* or to a lesser extent *T. tonsurans* which was responsible for many outbreaks in the UK in the 1960s, for example [16], and it was endemic at low levels in many countries, from Australia to Mexico [17].

Even though TC was brought under effective control at that time in Europe and North America after the introduction of griseofulvin and concerted public health interventions, the infection remained an endemic disease in some countries especially in Africa [1,18]. And also, it remained as a sporadic infection worldwide. Zoophilic TC was especially due to organisms like *M. canis* from cats or dogs, *T. mentagrophytes* from rodents, or *T. verrucosum* from cattle. Isolated occurrences of anthropophilic TC were due to organisms like *T. violaceum* from the Indian subcontinent [19].

In the last decades of the 20th century, some significant changes occurred with variations in the perceived prevalence of TC worldwide, where there was an overall increase once again in the number of cases of anthropophilic infections in children (especially *T. tonsurans* in the USA [20,21] and western European countries [1,22,23]), and *M. audouinii* and *T. soudanense* in France and the other European countries [24–27]. However, there was also an increase in the numbers of cases caused by zoophilic fungi such as *M. canis* [1].

In Africa, the incidence was considerably higher in countries such as Ethiopia with a fast and wide spread, this concerned mainly anthropophilic organisms reaching high prevalence rates (over 25% [28]), because there was no surveillance or any regular access to treatment except for severe cases due to organisms like *T. violaceum* and *T. schoenleinii* (favus). Also, a spread of organisms, in particular *T. tonsurans*, was also noticed [1,15].

Despite this upsurge of infection caused by anthropophilic fungi, no idea was confirmed if the outbreak was caused by new organisms, or whether there has been a resurgence of infection caused by the original strains, and when paediatric formulations of griseofulvin were difficult to obtain at that time, and also, there were a concern because *T. tonsurans* infections seemed to respond poorly to griseofulvin [24]. Preparations of new antifungal agents, such as terbinafine, itraconazole and fluconazole, have been approved for this indication in a few countries [1].

Currently, TC is still a common infection worldwide [10], and as known before, dermatophyte fungi most likely to cause TC vary from geographic region to region, and it may change with time, with introduction of new organisms in some areas by migration or immigration worldwide [15,29–31]. However, there is no evidence of a change in the virulence of the organisms. In recent years, the incidence rate of TC fluctuated and increased. In the past two decades, the main changes in TC epidemiology have been the shift of the dermatophytes from anthropophilic to zoophilic species, and the rise of *M. canis* as the dominant agent in infections in some parts of Europe [10,30,32], Argentina [33] and China

[4,6,34]. In addition, there was a spread of *T. tonsurans* again in urban communities in the USA [24], South America [35], Western Europe, UK [30], France [36], West Africa [37], and in other countries like Japan and Israel, the infection was found in different infected hosts mainly older children and adults [38,39].

Infections due to *T. violaceum* and *M. audouinii* were also reported in countries that were previously not endemic for these organisms [40,41].

In Africa, TC is still one of the most prevalent childhood health condition in some countries like Ethiopia [5], it affects over one in every four schoolchildren. Moreover, the most recent systematic review that investigated the burden of TC among children in Africa showed that the prevalence of TC was 23% (95% CI, 17%–29%) mostly caused by *Trichophyton* species. Over 96% of cases occur in sub-Saharan Africa alone, mainly Nigeria and Ethiopia. Also this study showed that there was a large discrepancy between the clinical and mycological diagnosis [2]. For instance, in a study of TC in Nigeria, *T. rubrum*, *T. mentagrophytes* followed by *M. canis* were the most prevalent organisms, while *T. tonsurans* was rare, as only one case was described. Risk factors significantly associated with the infection were family history of TC, age under 10 years, playing with animals, the sharing of combs and not bathing with soap [5,42].

In the north of Africa, available data are not homogeneous even within countries. In general, there was a decrease in the frequency of anthropophilic species, in favour of zoophilic species. In Morocco [1,2], *M. canis*, and *T. violaceum* were the main identified species [43,44]. *M. canis* was also the major causative agent in a study in Algeria in addition to *T. mentagrophytes* [45].

Tinea capitis favosa, caused by anthropophilic species (mainly *T. schoenleinii*), has significantly decreased worldwide, except for few cases detected in some countries such as China, Nigeria and Iran [10,12]. This infection is most frequently seen in children mainly boys between the age of 6 and 10; however, if not treated, favus may persist for life. The mean disease duration is approximately 5 years (10 days to 59 years) [12], and it is one of the differential diagnosis of scarring alopecia [10].

11.1.3 Risk Factors Associated with Tinea Capitis

The reasons for this increase in the incidence of TC are not clear. It may be due to a combination of many factors, mainly low socioeconomic status, high population densities and poor health practices [2,46].

Currently, neglected children living in the rural mountainous region have a great risk of infection especially for inflammatory TC (kerion). Other environmental and host-specific risk factors have been identified:

- *Age*: TC can affect all ages [7]; however, children between 1 and 8 years are more susceptible to this infection whatever their ethnic background [6], while infants and newborns are rarely affected [47–50]. TC is also rare in puberty; this may be explained by the fact that the triglycerides contained in sebum exert a fungistatic effect [51]. In addition, in adults, it affects mainly old patients [52,53], or patients with topical immunosuppressive treatments who usually have a modified clinical appearance [54], which is currently called tinea incognito [55].

- Ethnicity was also incriminated since there was evidence that the spread of some microorganisms such as *T. tonsurans* predominantly in black children [56–58].

- *Gender*: Sexual predilection varies depending on the causative dermatophytes. For instance, *Trichophyton* infections will affect both sexes equally during the childhood years. *M. canis* affects boys more than girls [6,13]. In general, boys were found to be at greater risk [3,59], and adults hosts were mainly females in previous publications [39,52].

- History of animal contact is a risk factor for zoophilic dermatophyte infection, especially *M. canis* [60] in children. However, adult hosts were more likely than children to have a history of infection with anthropophilic organisms [3,59].

- *Other Factors*: The hair type or hair styling could also play a role in determining the pattern of infection in each community. Another factor is the greater virulence of some organisms in particular climates, and also the reduced awareness or difficulties in maintaining adequate surveillance in some countries [1].

11.1.4 Tinea Capitis in Adults

Epidemiological and mycological characteristics in adult TC are different from those of children in terms of annual incidence, sex distribution and isolated dermatophytes. It is also less common; however, there has been an increase in its incidence [10,61], especially in postmenopausal women [62]. Proposed causative factors include hormonal disorders, immunosuppression, autoinoculation and transmission from affected children [13,63]. TC in adults is known to have unusual clinical findings, and can be initially misdiagnosed [10,63]. It is usually caused by anthropophilic fungi [15,63], and fungal species that are rather uncommon in children (*T. rubrum*) [62,64]. However, in recent studies in southeastern Korea and China [62], *M. canis* was among the most common dermatophytes. *T. violaceum*, *T. mentagrophytes* and *T. rubrum* were also frequent [52,62].

Also, *T. tonsurans* TC has become a growing epidemiological concern especially in adults with a different profile; it affects mainly young men [39]. Fortunately, oral terbinafine was found to be highly effective in TC due to this fungi; however, concomitant tinea corporis increased the risk for treatment failure [39].

11.1.5 Tinea Capitis Incognito

Tinea incognito in general is a dermatophytic infection whose clinical appearance is modified by topical or systemic steroids; it can mimic other skin diseases. TC incognito is not very common (5.4% in a study performed in Iran [55]). Its etiological agents are consistent with those of the general population, mainly *T. verrucosum* and *T. mentagrophytes* [55].

11.1.6 Epidemiology of TC and Clinical Varieties

The range of clinical expression of TC is broad, and depends on the causal agent, as well as the host's immune response. The diagnosis could be sometimes challenging since the clinical manifestations are variable, from asymptomatic scattered areas of individual hair loss with mild scaling to severe and inflammatory lesions with pustular plaques (kerion), and a possible extensive alopecia [15,24,57]. In addition, the infection could be asymptomatic, but those children with no signs may carry the organism and act as sources of infection to other children. Also, anthropophilic infections may mimic a wide variety of other scalp conditions [1].

In general, a pronounced inflammatory reaction is often seen in zoophilic infections or those spread from animals to human; by contrast in others, particularly those with anthropophilic dermatophytosis spread from human to human, lesions are often non-inflammatory and persistent [15]. It is still not clear whether this clinical nuance reflects the level of immunological responsiveness to these infections and the probable underlying predisposition especially in patients with other scalp or systemic disorders under immunosuppressive treatments [13,15].

Many species of dermatophytes are capable of invading hair shafts, whereas *Epidermophyton floccosum* and *Trichophyton concentricum* do not cause TC. All dermatophytes causing scalp ringworm can invade smooth or glabrous skin, and some can penetrate nails as well (*T. soudanense*) [15].

Clinical features depend on the causative organism; however, the clinical picture alone does not allow for definitive dermatophyte identification. Nevertheless, diagnostic clues may be obtained by dermatoscopy, Wood's lamp and microscopic evaluation of the shape of the spores; and their location in relation to the hair [10,29].

There are three main types of hair shaft invasion that, in part, determine the clinical presentation:

- *The ectothrix form*: This is characterized by arthrospores forming a sheath around the hair shaft that is invaded at the level of mid-follicle. The intrapilary hyphae grow down towards the bulb of the hair. Dermatophytes that typically cause ectothrix infections are *Microsporum* species such as *M. canis* and *M. audouinii* (small spores, "microsporosis") as well as *T. mentagrophytes* and *T. verrucosum* (large spores). Clinical appearance in ectothrix infections is characterized by scaly and inflamed plaques with hair loss and hair shafts breaking 2–3 mm or more above the scalp level.

- *The endothrix form*: This is marked by the dermatophyte invading the hair shaft without destroying the cuticle, it may be caused by anthropophilic species (in particular, *T. tonsurans*, *T. violaceum*, *T. soudanense* and *T. rubrum* [rare]). Endothrix infections are only weakly immunogenic and are merely associated with pityriasiform scaling of the scalp with or without mild erythema, the main clinical appearance is small black dots in the follicular ostia due to trichomalacia, the remaining hairs are filled with spores and have an intact cuticle. This is why, affected individuals could become asymptomatic carriers who may then transmit the infection to others [10,15].

  - Inflammatory TC is generally due to deep invasion of hair follicles by zoophilic dermatophytes such as *T. verrucosum*, *T. mentagrophytes*, *Trichophyton benhamiae*, or the geophilic organism (*M. gypseum*), causing follicular pustules that can evolve to massive purulent discharge (kerion) [65]. However, there have been recent reports in urban areas of inflammatory endothrix infections caused by *T. tonsurans* or *T. violaceum* in particular [10,15].

  - Microsporosis sensu stricto is an exception of a deep folliculitis that is not associated with any significant immunological response or abscess formation or clinical inflammatory erythema within the alopecic patches; it is usually caused by *M. audouinii* (anthropophilic) or *M. canis* (zoophilic) [10].

  - Favus: The favic type of infection is caused by the anthropophilic dermatophyte *T. schoenleinii*. Fungal hyphae form large clusters with yellowish cup-shaped crusts at the base of hairs where they enter the follicle at the level of the epidermis; the affected hairs may continue to grow, as it is less damaged [15]; and scarring atrophic alopecic patches are found in long-standing cases [15].

11.2 Conclusion

TC is no longer regarded as a health priority, even though it is still sporadic worldwide and endemic in some countries in Africa, where it is highly neglected and under-reported [2]. Also, the rise of *M. canis* as the dominant agent in infections in many countries should be worrisome, as *Microsporum* infections in children are known to have low cure rates to systemic drugs especially terbinafine [10,15,66]. Thus, efforts need to be performed with increased surveillance in schools coupled with prompt treatment of cases in humans, and their animals as well as screening within their families and their environment.

References

1. Hay RJ. Endemic scalp ringworm: an object lesson in control of a common fungal infection. *Curr Opin Infect Dis*. 2001;14(2):121–2.
2. Bongomin F, Olum R, Nsenga L, et al. Estimation of the burden of tinea capitis among children in Africa. *Mycoses*. 2021;64(4):349–63.
3. Cai W, Huang J, Li J, et al. Epidemiology and clinical findings of tinea capitis: a 23-year retrospective, single-center study in Guangzhou, China. *Mycopathologia*. 2023;188(5):507–514. doi: 10.1007/s11046-023-00730-4.
4. Wang X, Abuliezi R, Hasimu H, Zhang L, Abliz P. Retrospective Analysis of Tinea Capitis in Xinjiang, China. *Mycopathologia*. 2023;188(5):523–529. doi: 10.1007/s11046-022-00702-0
5. Birhanu MY, Temesgen H, Ketema DB, et al. Tinea capitis among school children in Ethiopia: a systematic review and meta analysis. *PLOS ONE*. 2023;18(2):e0280948.
6. Xiao YY, Zhou YB, Chao JJ, et al. Epidemiology of tinea capitis in children in Beijing and adjacent regions, China: a 15-year retrospective study. *Mycopathologia*. 2022.
7. Aharaz A, Jemec GBE, Hay RJ, et al. Tinea capitis asymptomatic carriers: what is the evidence behind treatment? *J Eur Acad Dermatol Venereol* 2021;35(11):2199–207.
8. de Hoog GS, Dukik K, Monod M, et al. Toward a novel multilocus phylogenetic taxonomy for the dermatophytes. *Mycopathologia*. 2017;182(1–2):5–31.
9. Bassiri-Jahromi S. Epidemiological trends in zoophilic and geophilic fungi in Iran. *Clin Exp Dermatol*. 2013;38(1):13–19.
10. Mayser P, Nenoff P, Reinel D, et al. S1 guidelines: tinea capitis. *J Dtsch Dermatol Ges J Ger Soc Dermatol* 2020;18(2):161–79.
11. Nenoff P, Handrick W, Krüger C, et al. Dermatomycoses due to pets and farm animals: neglected infections?. *Hautarzt Z Dermatol Venerol Verwandte Geb*. 2012;63(11):848–58.
12. Ilkit M. Favus of the scalp: an overview and update. *Mycopathologia*. 2010;170(3):143–54.
13. Al Aboud AM, Crane JS. Tinea capitis. In: *StatPearls 2023*. National Center for Biotechnology Information. Treasure Island, FL: StatPearls Publishing; 2023 [accessed 31 July 2023].
14. Chen XQ, Yu J. Global demographic characteristics and pathogen spectrum of tinea capitis. *Mycopathologia*. 2023;188(5):433-447. doi: 10.1007/s11046-023-00710-8.
15. Hay RJ. Tinea capitis: current status. *Mycopathologia* 2017;182(1–2):87–93.
16. Mackenzie DWR, Rusk LW. The mycological diagnostic service: a five-year survey (1959–1963). *Ulster Med J* 1964;33(2):94–100.
17. Kane J, Leavitt E, Summerbell RC, et al. An outbreak of *Trichophyton tonsurans* dermatophytosis in a chronic care institution for the elderly. *Eur J Epidemiol* 1988;4(2):144–9.

18. Verhagen AR. Distribution of dermatophytes causing tinea capitis in Africa. *Trop Geogr Med*. 1974;26(2):101–20.

19. Clayton YM. The changing pattern of tinea capitis in London schoolchildren. *Mykosen Suppl*. 1978;1:104–7.

20. Wilmington M, Aly R, Frieden IJ. *Trichophyton tonsurans* tinea capitis in the San Francisco Bay area: increased infection demonstrated in a 20-year survey of fungal infections from 1974 to 1994. *J Med Vet Mycol* 1996 Jul–Aug;34(4):285–7.

21. Howard R, Frieden IJ. Tinea capitis: new perspectives on an old disease. *Semin Dermatol* 1995;14(1):2–8.

22. Timen A, Bovée L, Leentvaar-Kuijpers A, et al. Tinea capitis in primary school age children in southeastern Amsterdam: primarily due to *Trichophyton tonsurans*. *Ned Tijdschr Geneeskd*. 1999;143(1):24–7.

23. Viguie-Vallanet C, Savaglio N, Piat C, et al. Epidemiology of *Microsporum langeronii* tinea capitis in the Paris suburban area. Results of 2 school and familial surveys. *Ann Dermatol Venereol*. 1997;124(10):696–9.

24. Elewski BE. Tinea capitis: a current perspective. *J Am Acad Dermatol* 2000;42(1):1–20.

25. Cremer G, Bousseloua N, Roudot-Thoraval F, et al. Tinea capitis in Creteil. Trends over ten years. *Ann Dermatol Venereol* 1998;125(3):171–3.

26. Williams JV, Honig PJ, McGinley KJ, et al. Semiquantitative study of tinea capitis and the asymptomatic carrier state in inner-city school children. *Pediatrics* 1995;96(2 Pt 1):265–7.

27. Hay RJ, Clayton YM, De Silva N, et al. Tinea capitis in south-east London-a new pattern of infection with public health implications. *Br J Dermatol* 1996;135(6):955–8.

28. Figueroa JI, Hawranek T, Abraha A, et al. Tinea capitis in south-western Ethiopia: a study of risk factors for infection and carriage. *Int J Dermatol* 1997;36(9):661–6.

29. Vargas-Navia N, Ayala Monroy GA, Franco Rúa C, et al. Tinea capitis in children. *Rev Chil Pediatr* 2020;91(5):773–83.

30. Fuller LC. Changing face of tinea capitis in Europe. *Curr Opin Infect Dis*. 2009;22:115–8.

31. Hay RJ, Robles W, Midgley G, et al. European confederation of medical mycology working party on tinea capitis. Tinea capitis in Europe: new perspective on an old problem. *J Eur Acad Dermatol Venereol*. 2001;15:229–33.

32. Charpantidis S, Siopi M, Pappas G, et al. Changing epidemiology of tinea capitis in Athens, Greece: the impact of immigration and review of literature. *J Fungi Basel Switz*. 2023;9(7):703.

33. Messina F, Walker L, Romero M de LM, et al. Tinea capitis: clinical features and therapeutic alternatives. *Rev Argent Microbiol*. 2021;53(4):309–13.

34. Zhi H, Shen H, Zhong Y, et al. Tinea capitis in children: a single-institution retrospective review from 2011 to 2019. *Mycoses*. 2021;64(5):550–4.

35. Sidrim JJ, Rocha MF, Leite JJ, et al. *Trichophyton tonsurans* strains from Brazil: phenotypic heterogeneity, genetic homology, and detection of virulence genes. *Can J Microbiol*. 2013;59:754–60.

36. Alshawa K, Lacroix C, Benderdouche M, et al. Increasing incidence of *Trichophyton tonsurans* in Paris, France: a 15-year retrospective study. *Br J Dermatol*. 2012;166: 1149–50.

37. Hogewoning AA, Adegnika AA, Bouwes Bavinck JN, et al. Prevalence and causative fungal species of tinea capitis among schoolchildren in Gabon. *Mycoses*. 2011;54:e354–9.

38. Sei Y. 2011 Epidemiological survey of dermatomycoses in Japan. *Med Mycol J*. 2015;56(4):J129–35.

39. Galili E, Goldsmith T, Khanimov I, et al. Tinea capitis caused by *Trichophyton tonsurans* among adults: clinical characteristics and treatment response. *Mycoses*. 2023;66(2):144–9.

40. Kieliger S, Glatz M, Cozzio A, et al. Tinea capitis and tinea faciei in the Zurich area - an 8-year survey of trends in the epidemiology and treatment patterns. *J Eur Acad Dermatol Venereol*. 2015;29(8):1524–9.

41. Mapelli ETM, Cerri A, Bombonato C, et al. Tinea capitis in the paediatric population in Milan, Italy: the emergence of *Trichophyton violaceum*. *Mycopathologia*. 2013;176(3–4):243–6.

42. Adesiji YO, Omolade FB, Aderibigbe IA, et al. Prevalence of tinea capitis among children in Osogbo, Nigeria, and the associated risk factors. *Dis Basel Switz*. 2019;7(1):13.

43. El Mezouari E, Hocar O, Atarguine H, et al. Tinea capitis in the military hospital Avicenna (Morocco): review of 8 years (2006–2013)]. *J Mycol Medicale*. 2016;26(1):e1–5.

44. Elmaataoui A, Zeroual Z, Lyagoubi M, et al. Profil étiologique des teignes du cuir chevelu à l'hôpital Ibn Sina de Rabat (Maroc). *J Mycol Médicale*. 2012;22(3):261–4.
45. Kheffache H, Seklaoui N, Bouchara JP, et al. Tinea capitis at the university hospital of Tizi-Ouzou, Algeria, and first isolation of *Trichophyton tonsurans*. *J Mycol Medicale*. 2020;30(4):101040.
46. Hay RJ, Johns NE, Williams HC, et al. The global burden of skin disease in 2010: an analysis of the prevalence and impact of skin conditions. *J Invest Dermatol*. 2014;134(6):1527–34.
47. Larralde M, Gomar N, Boggio P et al. Neonatal kerion Celsi: report of three cases. *Pediatr Dermatol*. 2010 Jul–Aug;27(4):361–3.
48. Atanasovski M, El Tal AK, Hamzavi F, et al. Neonatal dermatophytosis: report of a case and review of the literature: neonatal dermatophytosis. *Pediatr Dermatol*. 2011;28(2):185–8.
49. Zampella JG, Kwatra SG, Blanck J, et al. Tinea in Tots: cases and literature review of oral anti-fungal treatment of Tinea capitis in children under 2 years of age. *J Pediatr*. 2017;183:12–18.e3.
50. Fremerey C, Nenoff P. Tinea capitis in a newborn. *N Engl J Med*. 2018;378(21):2022.
51. Rothman S, Smiljanic A. The spontaneous cure of tinea capitis in puberty. *J Invest Dermatol*. 1947;8(2):81–98.
52. Lee HJ, Kim JY, Park KD, et al. Analysis of adult patients with tinea capitis in Southeastern Korea. *Ann Dermatol*. 2020;32(2):109–14.
53. Lahouel M, Mokni S, Chouaieb H, et al. Two erratic cases of tinea capitis in adults: utility of trichoscopy. *Int J Trichology*. 2020;12(3):118–20.
54. Sato Y, Shigeeda S, Ishizali S et al. A case of tinea capitis with a couple of nodular lesions possibly resulting from topical application of tacrolimus. *Nihon Ishinkin Gakkai Zasshi/Jpn J Med Mycol*. 2004;45(3):177–80.
55. Ansar A, Farshchian M, Nazeri H, et al. Clinico-epidemiological and mycological aspects of tinea incognito in Iran: a 16-year study. *Med Mycol J*. 2011;52(1):25–32.
56. Tack DA, Fleishcer, Jr A, McMichael A, et al. The epidemic of tinea capitis disproportionately affects school-aged African Americans. *Pediatr Dermatol*. 1999;16(1):75–75.
57. Child F, Higgins, DV. A study of the spectrum of skin disease occurring in a black population in south-east London. *Br J Dermatol*. 1999;141(3):512–7.
58. Williams HC, Burney PGJ, Hay RJ, et al. The UK working party's diagnostic criteria for atopic dermatitis. I. Derivation of a minimum set of discriminators for atopic dermatitis. *Br J Dermatol*. 1994;131:383–96.
59. Zheng D, Liang T, Wu W, et al. The epidemiology of tinea capitis in Guangxi Province, China. *Mycopathologia*. 2023.
60. Chen XQ, Zheng DY, Xiao YY, et al. Aetiology of tinea capitis in China: a multicentre prospective study. *Br J Dermatol*. 2022;186(4):705–12.
61. Binder B, Lackner HK, Poessl BD et al. Prevalence of tinea capitis in Southeastern Austria between 1985 and 2008: up-to-date picture of the current situation. *Mycoses*. 2011;54(3):243–7.
62. Liang G, Zheng X, Song G, et al. Adult tinea capitis in China: a retrospective analysis from 2000 to 2019. *Mycoses*. 2020;63(8):876–88.
63. Duarte B, Galhardas C, Cabete J. Adult tinea capitis and tinea barbae in a tertiary Portuguese hospital: a 11-year audit. *Mycoses*. 2019;62(11):1079–83.
64. Ziemer A, Kohl K, Schröder G. Trichophyton rubrum-induced inflammatory tinea capitis in a 63-year-old man. *Mycoses*. 2005;48(1):76–9.
65. Zhang R, Ran Y, Dai Y, A case of kerion celsi caused by *Microsporum gypseum* in a boy following dermatoplasty for a scalp wound from a road accident. *Med Mycol*. 2011;49(1):90–3.
66. Gupta AK, Talukder M, Carviel JL, Cooper EA, Piguet V. Combatting antifungal resistance: paradigm shift in the diagnosis and management of onychomycosis and dermatomycosis. *J Eur Acad Dermatol Venereol*. 2023;37(9):1706–1717. doi: 10.1111/jdv.19217.

12

Anatomy of the Scalp

Julia Nowowiejska, Giuseppe Argenziano, Anna Balato, and Vincenzo Piccolo

The scalp is limited by the external occipital protuberance and superior nuchal lines at the back, the supraorbital margins at the front [1] and both ears on the lateral parts [2]. Scalp consists of five layers. The uppermost layer is skin, right beneath there is subcutaneous tissue, galea aponeurotica, subgaleal space and the deepest layer is the pericranium [3] (Figure 12.1). It is observed that in the central areas without muscles or fascia, the scalp is tight, and in the peripheral areas where they are present, the scalp is rather loose [4].

The function of the scalp encompasses the protection against trauma or infections, thermoregulation and aesthetic aspects [5].

12.1 Skin

Skin is the most external part of the scalp. It consists of the epidermis, made of stratified squamous epithelium, and the dermis, made of fibrous connective tissue [6]. This layer includes hair, sebaceous and sweat glands [3]. The epidermis is an avascular layer, whereas the dermis includes blood vessels [6].

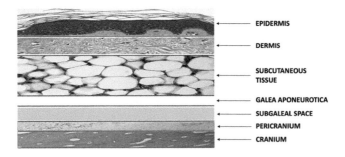

FIGURE 12.1
Scalp anatomy.

DOI: 10.1201/9781003381648-14

12.2 Subcutaneous Tissue (Hypodermis)

Subcutaneous tissue consists mainly of adipose tissue. It extends to the neck at the back, to temporalis muscles on the sides and bridge of the nose, and it blends with the adipose tissue above the orbicularis oculi and frontalis muscles [2]. The thickness of this layer may be dependent on the patient, e.g. it can be very thin in case of slim individuals [2].

12.3 Galea Aponeurotica (Epicranial Aponeurosis)

Galea is an unflexible dense membrane that lies beneath the hypodermis and above the subgaleal space [3]. Galea is a part of the subcutaneous musculoaponeurotic system (SMAS) [4]. It is possible that in some individuals it may be congenitally absent [2]. In the sagittal section, it extends between the occipital and frontal bellies of the occipito-frontalis muscles [3]. In the frontal section, it connects with the temporal fascia on both sides [3]. Galea blends with several muscles. At the front, the galea is associated with the paired frontalis muscle of the forehead. At the back, it blends with the paired occipitalis muscles. On the lateral sides, the galea is connected with the paired temporoparietalis muscles [2].

The first three layers – skin, hypodermis and galea – are considered a single unit due to their tight fitting [1].

12.4 Subgaleal Space (Merkel Space)

Subgaleal space is located beneath the galea aponeurotica and above the pericranium. It contains only a loose fibroareolar tissue, with no blood vessels [3]. This space is not present in the whole scalp area but extends from the superior nuchal lines and goes front to the forehead [3]. Inferiorly, it is adjacent to the superficial layer of the deep cervical fascia and to the temporal fascia and temporal muscles on the lateral parts [7]. Subgaleal space provides the scalp the ability to be moved freely in some parts and is responsible for scalp laxity [4].

12.5 Pericranium (Periosteum)

Pericranium is the deepest part of the scalp which directly covers the skull and is located beneath the subgaleal space. Pericranium is made of dense connective tissue [5] and is loosely attached to the galea but very tightly to the cranial sutures [3,8]. It contains an extensive vascular network [4].

12.6 Scalp Blood, Lymph and Nerve Supply

Arterial supply comes with the arteries: superficial temporal, occipital, supratrochlear, supraorbital and posterior auricular, which go within the hypodermis [4].

There are no lymph nodes in the scalp area; however, there are lymphatic vessels, located below the dermis or hypodermis that drain towards the parotid glands, preauricular and retroauricular areas, the upper part of the neck and occipital region [4].

The nerve supply consists of motor, sensory and autonomic fibres [2]. The first branch of the trigeminal nerve, ophthalmic nerve, provides sensory fibres to the anterior part of the scalp through the supraorbital and supratrochlear nerves. The lesser occipital nerve, a branch of the cervical plexus, innervates the posterior part of the scalp. Sensory innervation in the temporal region is provided by the auriculotemporal nerve [4]. The motor innervation of the mimic muscles is provided by the facial nerve [2].

12.7 Hair

Hair consists of the hair follicle and the hair shaft [9]. It is anchored within the subcutaneous tissue but extends up through the dermis and epidermis to the external surface of the scalp [9].

The hair shaft consists of the medulla, cortex and cuticle [10]. The medulla is the central structure in the hair shaft, whereas the cortex and the cuticle are located outside the medulla and play an important role in the physical endurance and resistance of the hair to external stimuli [9].

The hair follicle is composed of the outer and inner root sheath [9]. The outer root sheath is a source of multipotent stem cells and keratinocytes [9]. A very important structure that is formed by the outer sheath is the bulge area. It is located between the insertion of the arrector pili muscle and the sebaceous gland duct [9]. The inner root sheath separates the hair shaft from the outer root sheath and consists of the cuticle, Huxley's layer and Henle's layer [9, 10]. The role of this sheath is to attach the hair shaft to the hair follicle [9].

The hair bulb is a part of the hair follicle [9] which contains hair matrix and follicular papilla [10]. Its role is hair production [9]. The bulb is divided into two parts by so-called Auber's line – upper and lower [9]. The lower part is composed of undifferentiated cells and contains matrix and dermal papilla [9]. The upper region contains cells that become differentiated [9]. In this part, four others are distinguished: pre-elongation region, cellular elongation region, cortical pre-keratinization region and the last is the keratogenous zone [9]. Above the hair bulb, there are two essential structures observed – the infundibulum and the isthmus [9]. The infundibulum goes from the scalp surface to the sebaceous gland duct and contains sebum [9]. The isthmus, on the other hand, goes from the sebaceous gland duct to the exertion of the arrector pili muscle [9].

The hair possesses blood and nerve supply. The arteries come from the hypodermis through the dermis and form a plexus, especially gathered around the lower region of the hair follicle [9]. Of note, the vessel arrangement can change during the particular phases of the hair cycle [9]. As for the nerve supply, the hair follicle contains sensory afferent fibres, as well as autonomic sympathetic nerves, which originate in the dermis or hypodermis [9].

On the whole scalp, there are about 100,000? hair follicles. The hair undergoes a cycle of specific changes. The hair cycle is divided into three stages: anagen, catagen and telogen. The first phase – anagen – is the growth stage. It lasts a few years and it involves the majority of hair on the scalp. The second phase – catagen – is a transitional stage. It lasts a few weeks. The third stage – telogen – is the resting phase and it involves about 10% of all hair. It lasts a few weeks to months [9].

12.8 Sebaceous Glands

Sebaceous glands are located within the dermis and epidermis and are connected to the upper part of the hair follicle – below the infundibulum and above the bulge area and isthmus [11]. They are holocrine-type glands [12] which are associated with their anatomy. At the basal cell layer, there are proliferative cells located, and inside the gland, there are the sebocytes that contain lipids, and it is their breakdown that causes the production of the sebum [11]. Indeed, the primary function of the sebaceous glands is sebum secretion but besides that, they are considered to exert neuroendocrine and immunological properties [12]. Sebum plays several essential roles: it moistures the skin which translates into its elasticity, takes part in thermoregulation, constitutes a protective barrier against pathogens or modulates the interplay between the commensal and pathogenic microbiota [12].

12.9 Sweat Glands

In general, there are two types of sweat glands: eccrine and apocrine. On the scalp, there are only eccrine sweat glands present [13]. They are composed of two parts: a coiled secretory region located in the dermis or hypodermis, and a straight or helical ductular part that extends to the skin surface [13]. The main role of sweat glands is thermoregulation. However, sweat also may exert a protective influence against pathogens due to the content of urea, lactate or immunoglobulins [13].

The microenvironment of the scalp containing hair follicles and significant sebum secretion contributes to the risk of fungal infections [5].

References

1. Dong J, Gong X, Gao W, et al. The "Hand as Foot" teaching method in scalp anatomy and hematoma. *Asian J Surg*. 2023;46(2):1124–5.
2. Hayman LA, Shukla V, Ly C, et al. Clinical and imaging anatomy of the scalp. *J Comput Assist Tomogr*. 2003;27(3):454–9.

3. Seery GE. Surgical anatomy of the scalp. *Dermatol Surg.* 2002;28(7):581–7.
4. Earnest LM, Byrne PJ. Scalp reconstruction. *Facial Plast Surg Clin North Am.* 2005;13(2):345–53.
5. Tajran J, Gosman AA. Anatomy, head and neck, scalp. [Updated 2023 Jul 24]. In: *StatPearls* [Internet]. Treasure Island, FL: StatPearls Publishing; 2024 Jan-. https://www.ncbi.nlm.nih.gov/books/NBK551565/
6. Arda O, Göksügür N, Tüzün Y. Basic histological structure and functions of facial skin. *Clin Dermatol.* 2014;32(1):3–13.
7. Sittitavornwong S, Morlandt AB. Reconstruction of the scalp, calvarium, and frontal sinus. *Oral Maxillofac Surg Clin North Am.* 2013;25(2):105–29.
8. Hacking C, Bell D, Baba Y, et al. *Scalp. Reference article*, Radiopaedia.org (Accessed on 03 Oct 2023). Available from: https://doi.org/10.53347/rID-52595
9. Buffoli B, Rinaldi F, Labanca M, et al. The human hair: from anatomy to physiology. *Int J Dermatol.* 2014, 53(3):331–41.
10. Panteleyev AA. Functional anatomy of the hair follicle: the secondary hair germ. *Exp Dermatol.* 2018;27(7):701–20.
11. Niemann C, Horsley V. Development and homeostasis of the sebaceous gland. *Semin Cell Dev Biol.* 2012;23(8):928–36.
12. Picardo M, Mastrofrancesco A, Bíró T. Sebaceous gland – a major player in skin homoeostasis. *Exp Dermatol.* 2015;24(7):485–6.
13. Groscurth P. Anatomy of sweat glands. *Curr Probl Dermatol.* 2002;30:1–9.

13

Clinical Patterns Correlated with Routes of Entry for the Scalp

Michela Starace and Francesca Pampaloni

13.1 Involvement of the Length of the Hair Shaft

13.1.1 Piedra

The term "piedra", which means "stone" in Spanish, also known as Trichomycosis nodosa, reflects the fact that the fungal elements stick together to form nodules along the hair shaft. It is a superficial infection that starts under the hair cuticle and spreads outwards. It can lead to progressive weakening and breakage of the hair. Nodules can even envelop the hair shaft as they grow. The clinical appearance and microscopic findings distinguish the two main forms: black piedra and white piedra [1].

13.1.1.1 Black Piedra

In black piedra, the fungal elements are attached along the hair shaft to form nodules. It predominantly affects scalp hair, although involvement of the beard, moustache and pubic hairs is also described. Black piedra is common in hot and humid countries like South American countries and Southeast Asian countries. It is caused by a particular type of fungus called *Piedraia hortae*. This fungal disease results from poor personal hygiene. It is often seen in people with long hair and excessive use of various hair oils. Practices such as prolonged wearing of veils or tight hats may contribute to its development and progression [2,3]. The minute hair shaft nodules of black piedra can have a gritty feeling or be recognized by a metallic sound when brushing hair. This infection usually affects scalp hair, and findings can include darkly pigmented nodules that vary in size up to as large as a few millimetres in diameter.

13.1.1.2 White Piedra

Patients with white piedra manifest with soft, less adherent nodules that are typically white but may also be red, green or light brown in colour. White piedra is due mainly to fungi in the *Trichosporon* genus, class Basidiomycetes. *Trichosporon* genus includes six different human pathogenic species: *Trichosporon ovoides*, *Trichosporon inkin*, *Trichosporon mucoides* and *Trichosporon asahii* [4]. *Trichosporon* species most associated with white piedra are *T. ovoides* and *T. inkin*. *T. ovoides* mostly causes white piedra of the scalp, while *T. inkin* is restricted to the groin [5]. White piedra can be easily detached from the hair shaft because it affects the outer lipid layers.

DOI: 10.1201/9781003381648-15

13.2 Involvement of Base of the Hair Shaft

13.2.1 Dermatophytosis

Tinea capitis is a common dermatophyte infection of the scalp, and it affects the base of the hair shaft and the follicle, unlike piedra. Clinically, tinea capitis can be divided into inflammatory and non-inflammatory types. The non-inflammatory type usually will not be complicated by scarring alopecia. The inflammatory type may result in a kerion (see below), a painful nodule with pus, and scarring alopecia. Dermatophytes are a common cause of infection in humans. Once acquired, the fungus grows downwards in the stratum corneum and invades the keratin. The infected hair eventually becomes brittle and will then break. Immunosuppression may lead to impaired hair shaft growth and strength leading to easier colonization. Other associated diseases may include diabetes mellitus, prolonged steroid use, cancer, use of immunosuppressant medications.

Hair can be typically infected in one of three principal routes:

- *Endothrix*: Where the fungi affect the hair shaft
- *Ectothrix*: Where the fungi affect the outer sheath root
- *Favus*: Where there is an inflammatory reaction, crusting or scutula and hair loss

The causative pathogens are members of only two genera: *Trichophyton* and *Microsporum*. *Trichophyton tonsurans* is currently the most common cause of tinea capitis in the US (accounting for >90% of cases), with a predilection for individuals of African descent, and *Microsporum canis* is the second most frequent aetiology [6–10]. There are significant differences in the epidemiology of tinea capitis worldwide, and different clinical presentations arise from the various causative organisms.

13.2.2 Infection Outside the Hair Shaft

13.2.2.1 Ectothrix

The ectothrix pattern occurs when arthroconidia are formed from fragmented hyphae outside the hair shaft. Destruction of the cuticle occurs. The most common pathogens are: *M. canis*, *Microsporum audouinii*, *Microsporum ferrugineum*, *Microsporum distortum*, *Microsporum gypseum* and *Trichophyton rubrum* (rare). *M. audouinii* is the causative pathogen of ectothrix form of tinea capitis that typically presents with dry, scaly patches of alopecia ("grey patch" tinea capitis). Ectothrix infection can be fluorescent (*Microsporum*) or non-fluorescent (*Microsporum and Trichophyton*), as determined by Wood's lamp examination. Clinical features vary from patchy, scaly alopecia with little inflammation that may mimic alopecia areata to kerion formation [6,11] (see Figures 13.1–13.3).

13.2.3 Infection within the Hair Shaft

13.2.3.1 Endothrix

The endothrix pattern results from infection with anthropophilic fungi in the genus *Trichophyton* and is characterized by non-fluorescent arthroconidia within the hair shaft. *T. tonsurans* and *Trichophyton violaceum* are important causes of endothrix infection. Other less common pathogens are: *Trichophyton Soudanense*, *Trichophyton gourville*, *Trichophyton*

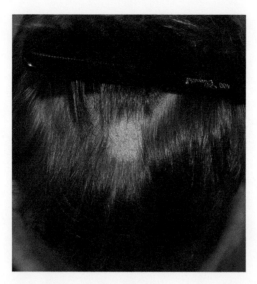

FIGURE 13.1
Clinical presentation of tinea capitis.

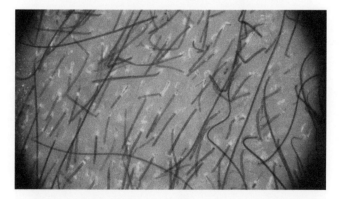

FIGURE 13.2
Trichoscopy of tinea capitis showing comma hair, Morse code hair and hair casts.

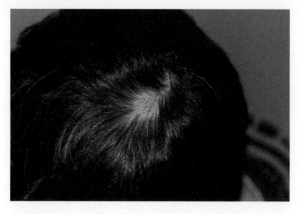

FIGURE 13.3
Clinical presentation of tinea capitis.

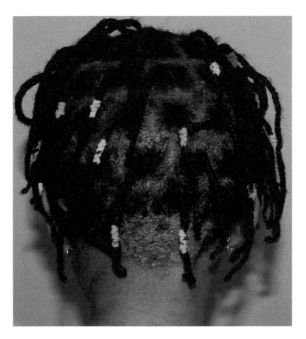

FIGURE 13.4
Clinical presentation of tinea capitis.

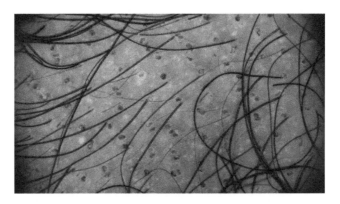

FIGURE 13.5
Trichoscopy of tinea capitis showing comma hair, zigzag hair, black dots and corkscrew hair.

yaoundei and *T. rubrum*. The clinical presentation varies from scaling to "black dots" due to hair breakage near the scalp with patchy alopecia to kerion formation [6] (see Figures 13.4 and 13.5).

13.2.3.2 Favus

Favus is the most severe form of dermatophyte hair infection and is most frequently caused by *Trichophyton schoenleinii*. *T. violaceum*, *Trichophyton verrucosum*, zoophilic *Trichophyton mentagrophytes* (referred to as "var. *quinckeanum*"), *M. canis* and geophilic *M. gypseum* have also been recovered from favic lesions. The characteristic type of hair invasion in favus (endothrix infection) contributes to the chronic course of the favus, which persists as long as there is hair. Tinea favosa usually occurs in children and adolescents and persists throughout adult life in the absence of treatment. It has an insidious course, without an acute phase, leading to the diagnosis delay [12,13]. In 95% of cases, favus begins with folliculocentric erythemato-squamous areas. If these lesions are removed, the scutulum starts to develop. The classic favus lesion is the "scutulum", a concave, cup-shaped yellow crust on the scalp centrally pierced by dull grey hair, with underlying erythema and glabrous skin that is associated with severe alopecia [13,14]. These keratotic crusts contain fungal hyphae and can be highly infectious. Hyphae and air spaces are observed within the hair shaft, and a bluish-white or bright green fluorescence by Wood's lamp examination is typically seen. Scarring alopecia may develop in chronic infections. Affected skin is characterized by a mousy or cheesy odour.

Secondary bacterial infections can occur with pus and lymphadenopathy [15]. As the disease progresses, many scutula coalesce to involve more than one-third of the scalp. Untreated, favus is classically slowly progressive. The parasitized hair can fall out, causing extensive permanent alopecia, atrophy and scarring.

The treatment outcome varies with the stage at which the condition is diagnosed. With early diagnosis and proper therapeutic management, favus can be cured without sequelae. However, late treatment leads to the ultimate scarring alopecia in all clinical presentations [16].

13.2.3.3 Kerion

Kerion celsi is an acute purulent inflammatory process of scalp, probably due to a T-cell-mediated hypersensitivity reaction to the dermatophyte. The lesion begins as a group of inflammatory follicular papules, gradually fusing into a protuberant inflammatory mass with a soft texture (Figures 13.6–13.8). The surface then transforms into honeycomb-shaped pus-discharging pores. Secondary bacterial infection leads to abscess formation. A kerion results from advanced disease coupled with an exaggerated host response that leads to boggy, purulent plaques with abscess formation and associated alopecia and scar formation. Some patients may even become systemically ill with extensive

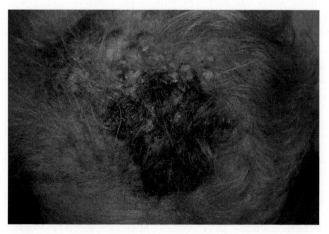

FIGURE 13.6
Clinical presentation of kerion.

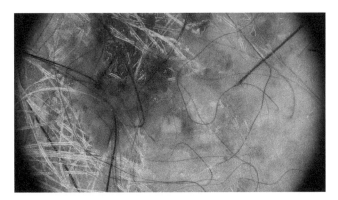

FIGURE 13.7
Trichoscopy of kerion showing follicular pustules.

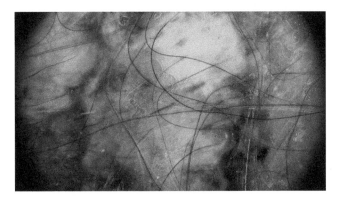

FIGURE 13.8
Trichoscopy of kerion showing confluent pustules.

lymphadenopathy. The hair in the affected area usually returns, but the longer the infection persists, the more likely the alopecia will be permanent [17]. The aetiological agents responsible for causing kerion are most commonly zoophilic dermatophytes such as *M. canis* and *T violaceum* [18], and an unusual case due to *Aspergillus protuberans* infection has been reported [19].

If a kerion is misdiagnosed as a bacterial abscess and treated with antibiotics following incision and drainage, the infection will likely worsen, thereby increasing the likelihood of scarring alopecia.

References

1. Schwartz RA. Superficial fungal infections. *Lancet*. 2004 Sep 25–Oct 1;364(9440):1173–82.
2. Desai DH, Nadkarni NJ. Piedra: an ethnicity-related trichosis? *Int J Dermatol*. 2014;53(8):1008–11.
3. Elewski BE, Hazen PG. The superficial mycoses and the dermatophytes. *J Am Acad Dermatol*. 1989 Oct;21(4 Pt 1):655–73.

4. Thérizol-Ferly M, Kombila M, Gomez de Diaz M, et al. White piedra and *Trichosporon* species in equatorial Africa. I. History and clinical aspects: an analysis of 449 superficial inguinal specimens. *Mycoses.* 1994;37(7–8):249–53.
5. Shivaprakash MR, Singh G, Gupta P et al. Extensive white piedra of the scalp caused by *Trichosporon* inkin: a case report and review of literature. *Mycopathologia.* 2011;172(6):481–6.
6. Leung AKC, Hon KL, Leong KF, et al. Tinea capitis: an updated review. *Recent Pat Inflamm Allergy Drug Discov.* 2020;14(1):58–68.
7. Al Aboud AM, Crane JS. Tinea Capitis. 2023 Aug 8. In: *StatPearls [Internet].* Treasure Island (FL): StatPearls Publishing; 2024 Jan–. PMID: 30725594.
8. Elghblawi E. Idiosyncratic findings in trichoscopy of tinea capitis: comma, zigzag hairs, corkscrew, and Morse code-like hair. *Int J Trichology.* 2016;8(4):180–3.
9. Fuller LC, Barton RC, Mohd Mustapa MF, et al. British Association of Dermatologists' guidelines for the management of tinea capitis 2014. *Br J Dermatol.* 2014;171(3):454–63.
10. John AM, Schwartz RA, Janniger CK. The kerion: an angry tinea capitis. *Int J Dermatol.* 2018; 57(1):3–9.
11. Auchus IC, Ward KM, Brodell RT, et al. Tinea capitis in adults. *Dermatol Online J.* 2016; 16;22(3). doi: 10.5070/d3223030362.
12. Zaraa I, Zaouek A, El Euch D, et al. Tinea capitis favosa in a 73-year-old immunocompetent Tunisian woman. *Mycoses.* 2012;55(5):454–6.
13. Ilkit M. Favus of the scalp: an overview and update. *Mycopathologia.* 2010;170(3):143–54.
14. Do N, Notaro E, Schillhammer G, et al. Tinea capitis mimicking favus in rural Washington state. *JAAD Case Rep.* 2020;6(3):187–188.
15. Poppe H, Kolb-Mäurer A, Wobser M, et al. Pitfall scarring alopecia: favus closely mimicking lichen planus. *Mycoses.* 2013;56(3):382–4.
16. Anane S, Chtourou O. Tinea capitis favosa misdiagnosed as tinea amiantacea. *Med Mycol Case Rep.* 2012 Dec 28;2:29–31.
17. Sonthalia S, Khurana R. Kerion. *Indian J Pediatr.* 2016 Jan;83(1):94–5. doi: 10.1007/s12098-015-1760-0. Epub 2015 May 8. PMID: 25947263.
18. Kudava K, Kituashvili T, Sekania M, et al. Some characteristics of tinea capitis. *Iran J Pediatr.* 2013;23(6):707–8.
19. Jia J, Chen M, Mo X, et al. The first case report of kerion-type scalp mycosis caused by *Aspergillus protuberans.* *BMC Infect Dis.* 2019;19(1):506.

14

Clinical Differential Diagnosis of Scalp Infection

Francesca Pampaloni, Michela Starace, and Bianca Maria Piraccini

14.1 Piedra

14.1.1 Black Piedra

Black piedra is characterized by black-coloured nodules along the hair shafts and is generally diagnosed by clinical and microscopic inspection of the hair. It must be distinguished from several different conditions causing areas of hair shaft swelling like: pediculosis (nits), hair casts, trichorrhexis nodosa, trichomycosis axillaris, psoriasis and eczema. Unlike eczema and psoriasis, the scalp typically appears normal in piedra.

- *Pediculosis Capitis*: Black piedra is often confused with pediculosis capitis because the lice eggs (nits) look similar to black piedra nodules. Nits are oval in shape and light grey, tan or yellowish in colour. They firmly attach to the hair shaft and are difficult to remove. Nits carrying viable eggs are close to the scalp. Diagnostic confirmation of head lice relies on the finding of viable eggs, nits in various stages (live and viable, open, empty/dead) or adult lice [1,2].

- *Trichorrhexis Nodosa*: It is an inherited or acquired disorder of the hair shaft characterized by fragility with easy breakage and nodes (swellings) on the hair shaft. The microscopic examination of the node reveals a fractured hair. At the point of fracture, there is visible splaying out and release of individual cortical cells that resemble two brooms facing each other [3].

- *Monilethrix*: It is a rare autosomal dominant hair disorder that results in fragile, broken hair that appears beaded. Under light microscopy, the hair shaft has regular elliptical, fusiform or spindle-shaped parts separated by constricted internodes devoid of medulla (Figure 14.1) [4].

- *Trichomycosis Axillaris*: It is an uncommon condition caused by *Corynebacterium tenuis* that forms opaque brown formations around the hair. The diagnosis is guided by the Wood's lamp examination, which shows yellowish-green fluorescence. Fungal and bacterial cultures readily differentiate white piedra by trichomycosis axillaris. Dermoscopic evaluation with non-contact polarized light dermoscopy shows sheaths around the hair with cotton-like structures [5,6].

Black and white piedra should always be distinguished. White piedra, unlike black piedra, more often occurs on the scalp hair and spares other hair. It is caused by *Trichosporon* spp. and manifests as whitish, loose adherent material on the scalp hair shafts. Trichoscopy and a fungal culture can easily distinguish the two conditions. The septate hyphae of *Trichosporon* causing white piedra are non-dematiaceous [2].

DOI: 10.1201/9781003381648-16

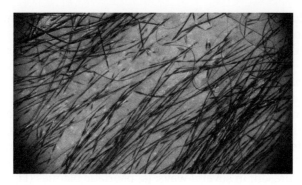

FIGURE 14.1
Trichoscopy of monilethrix: beaded fragile hair shafts.

14.2 Tinea Capitis

Different clinical presentations of tinea capitis have been described, resulting from different causative agents. The three main findings of tinea capitis are scaly patches with alopecia, alopecia with black dots or hair broken a few millimetres above the scalp and diffuse scalp scaling with subtle hair loss. Scalp scaling is a prominent feature of all types of tinea capitis. Hair shaft breakage occurs at the level of the scalp in endothrix infections or 1–3 mm from the scalp in ectothrix infections. Pustular lesions may be seen in inflammatory tinea capitis (kerion) [7].

Trichoscopy represents a fundamental tool for the diagnosis [8]. It can highlight:

- Comma hair with a curved C-shaped appearance (both ectothrix and endothrix infection);
- Broken hair with a constant diameter throughout their length;
- Black dots: rounded formations in correspondence of the follicular ostia due to breakage of the hair at the ostium level;
- Corkscrew hair: broken hair coiled in a corkscrew pattern visible in dark-coloured individuals;
- Scaling: diffuse and around the hair shafts (hair casts);
- Scalp erythema;
- Folliculitis as a non-specific sign of tinea capitis, which trap the broken hair inside the pustule.

KOH examination of the hair helps to differentiate ecto- and endothrix hair invasion. The cultural sample identifies the fungal species [9].

Histopathology shows a superficial and deep perifollicular infiltrate rich in neutrophils, eosinophils, lymphocytes and plasma cells. Periodic acid–Schiff (PAS) staining identifies the presence of hyphae and spores [8–10].

Tinea capitis can range from non-inflammatory scaling that resembles seborrheic dermatitis to a severe pustular reaction with alopecia, known as a kerion.

There are many scalp and hair disorders that cause scaling or alopecia (scarring and non-scarring) that are not caused by fungal infections. Fungal infection should always be considered and excluded in alopecia associated with scaling, especially in children and in post-menopausal women.

Main differential diagnosis of tinea capitis are as follows (Table 14.1):

- *Seborrheic Dermatitis*: It is a common scalp disorder that most frequently produces scalp scaling (dandruff) associated with mild erythema and itching and it can sometimes mimic the symptoms of tinea capitis. Trichoscopy of seborrheic dermatitis is characterized by fine white yellowish scales, orange-yellowish areas, dotted vessels in a patchy distribution and linear branching vessels (Figure 14.2) [11].
- *Psoriasis*: It can present in several ways: (a) psoriatic plaques (Figure 14.3), (b) thin scales, (c) psoriatic cap, (d) pityriasis amiantacea (Figure 14.4), (e) sebopsoriasis, (f) pustular psoriasis. Trichoscopy shows: white-silvery diffuse scales, erythema and an extremely typical vascular pattern characterized by red dots, globules and twisted loops, which are not found in tinea capitis (Figure 14.5) [12].

TABLE 14.1

Main Differential Diagnosis of Tinea Capitis

	Tinea Capitis	Seborrheic Dermatitis	Scalp Psoriasis	Contact Dermatitis	Alopecia Areata	Trichotillomania
Patches number	1 or more	1 or more	1 or more	Diffuse	1 or more	1
Shapes/ edge	Round/sharp	Irregular/blurred	Irregular/ sharp or blurred	Irregular/ blurred	Round/sharp	Irregular/blurred
Occurrence	Fast	Chronic recurrent	Chronic recurrent	Fast	Fast	Slow
Appearance	Broken hair and scales	Orange-yellowish areas with with/ yellow scales	Erythema and silvery-white scales	Diffuse erythema and scales	No hair and inflammatory signs	Hair of different lengths
Symptoms	Itchy	Itchy	Itchy	Itchy	None	None
Trichoscopy	Comma hair, broken hair, black dots, corkscrew hair, Morse code	Dotted vessels and fine white yellowish scales	White scales, red dots, globules and twisted loops	Scales, arborizing vessels, red loops	Black dots, yellow dots, exclamation mark hair	Broken, flam, hook hair

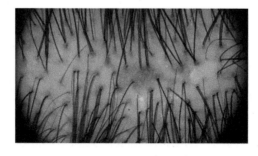

FIGURE 14.2
Trichoscopy of seborrheic dermatitis: white yellow scales and patchy erythematous areas.

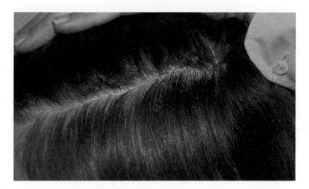

FIGURE 14.3
Scalp psoriasis presenting as diffuse thick scales.

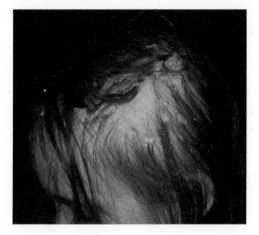

FIGURE 14.4
Pseudotinea amiantacea.

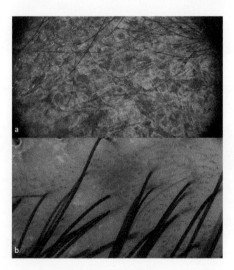

FIGURE 14.5
Trichoscopy of psoriasis: (a) magnification 20×: diffuse scaling and scalp erythema, (b) magnification 70×: regularly distributed dilated glomerular vessels, red haemorrhages.

- Contact dermatitis of the scalp is characterized by skin inflammation and irritation of the scalp due to contact with irritants or allergens. Erythema, diffuse scales and patchy scales are the main findings reported. Among the identified vascular patterns, the most described are arborizing vessels and simple red loops, while twisted red loops were less common [13].
- *Alopecia Areata*: It is an autoimmune condition that leads to hair loss in round patches on the scalp, with sharp margins and no signs of inflammation, which may initially appear similar to hair loss caused by tinea capitis (Figure 14.6a). Trichoscopy is useful to distinguish alopecia areata from tinea capitis, in particular in the paediatric population, where both diseases are very common. The main trichoscopic signs of alopecia areata are: (1) yellow dots that represent empty hair follicles; (2) black dots that represent broken hair shafts within the follicular ostium of hair loss and are commonly seen in acute alopecia areata; (3) exclamation mark hairs which are short, broken and tapered hair shafts that are wider at the top and thinner at the bottom; (4) short vellus hairs. No scales are usually detected in alopecia areata (Figure 14.6b) [14,15].
- Trichotillomania is characterized by the compulsive urge to pull out one's hair, leading to noticeable hair loss. The patches appear slowly, differently from tinea capitis. Patches are usually single, with bizarre shape and not itchy, with hair broken at different lengths (Figure 14.7a). Trichoscopic findings in trichotillomania are broken hair of different length, hook hair, frayed hair or split ends (short hair with trichoptilosis), tulip hairs (hair with hyperpigmented ends) and flame hairs (semi-transparent, wavy and redispersed conical hairs). Trichoscopy can also be useful to detect

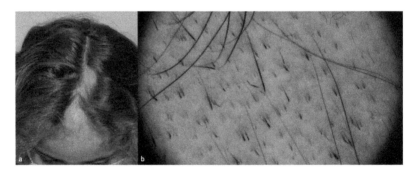

FIGURE 14.6
Patchy alopecia areata: (a) clinical presentation; (b) trichoscopy showing black dots, broken hairs and exclamation mark hairs.

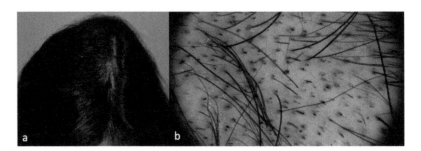

FIGURE 14.7
Trichotillomania: (a) clinical presentation; (b) trichoscopy showing hair broken at different length and clots of hair.

the V-sign, when two or more hairs emerge from the same follicle and are broken to the same length, and the presence of hair powder or clumps of hair (Figure 14.7b). Usually scaling is absent, and fungal cultures are negative [14,16].

Some more aggressive cases of scalp fungal infection, leading to kerion, must be distinguished from the following scalp disorders that cause scarring alopecia:

- Lichen planopilaris is a cicatricial alopecia characterized by one or multiple patches of alopecia with irregular shape and margins, frequently localized in the central scalp with intense itching. Pull test in active phase is positive with anagen roots surrounded by thick sheaths. Trichoscopy shows absence of follicular ostia, indicative of scarring alopecia, perifollicular erythema and hyperkeratosis (Figure 14.8) [14].
- Discoid lupus erythematosus (DLE) is a chronic, cicatricial, photosensitive dermatosis. It can present with one or few erythematous patches of pink to vivid red colour with skin atrophy, loss of follicular ostia, follicular plugging and adherent scales. Trichoscopic findings typical of DLE depend on the stage of the lesions: active lesions include yellow-brown dots and red dots, diffuse and follicular hyperkeratosis with follicular plugging, whereas long-standing inactive lesions show absence of follicular openings, cicatricial milky red or white patches, structureless white and brown areas, and thick arborizing vessels [14,17].
- Folliculitis decalvans is a neutrophilic cicatricial alopecia with chronic course characterized by relapsing of follicular pustular lesions leading to fibrosis and scarring. It is also called tufted folliculitis, as the presence of 10–15 hairs emerging from a single follicular opening is a diagnostic typical finding. A patch of hair loss with peripheral pustules, crusts and tufted hairs is commonly seen on the vertex and occipital area of the scalp. Bleeding, pain and burning sensation can be indicated by the patient (Figure 14.9) [18,19].
- Central centrifugal cicatricial alopecia is typical of dark-skinned population and begins in the central area of the scalp and has a progressive and symmetric centrifugal evolution. Trichoscopy shows peripilar grey/white halo that is a specific and sensitive sign; pinpoint white dots, hair shaft variability, white patches, perifollicular erythema, concentric white perifollicular and interfollicular scales, broken hairs, interfollicular-pigmented asterisk-like or stellate brown macules [20].

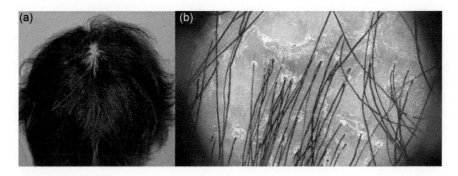

FIGURE 14.8
Lichen planopilaris: (a) clinical presentation; (b) trichoscopy showing areas without follicular ostia surrounded by follicular hyperkeratosis.

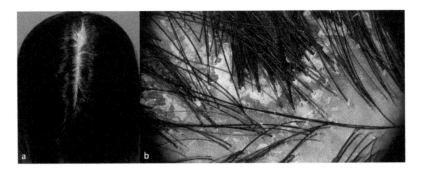

FIGURE 14.9
Folliculitis decalvans: (a) clinical presentation; (b) trichoscopy showing hair tufting and follicular pustules.

References

1. Desai DH, Nadkarni NJ. Piedra: an ethnicity-related trichosis? *Int J Dermatol.* 2014 Aug;53(8):1008–11. doi: 10.1111/j.1365-4632.2012.05722.x.
2. Elewski BE, Hazen PG. The superficial mycoses and the dermatophytes. *J Am Acad Dermatol.* 1989 Oct;21(4 Pt 1):655–73. doi: 10.1016/s0190-9622(89)70234-6.
3. Rudnicka L, Olszewska M, Waśkiel A, Rakowska A. Trichoscopy in hair shaft disorders. *Dermatol Clin.* 2018 Oct;36(4):421–30. doi: 10.1016/j.det.2018.05.009.
4. Chabchoub I, Souissi A. Monilethrix. 2023 Jun 12. In: *StatPearls [Internet].* Treasure Island, FL: StatPearls Publishing; 2024 Jan–. PMID: 30969635.
5. Murphy E, Maiberger M. Trichomycosis axillaris. *N Engl J Med.* 2022 Dec 1;387(22):e59. doi: 10.1056/NEJMicm2206453.
6. Almazán-Fernández FM, Fernández-Crehuet Serrano P. Trichomycosis axillaris dermoscopy. *Dermatol Online J.* 2017 Jun 15;23(6):13030/qt5hp5x1kz.
7. Schwartz RA. Superficial fungal infections. *Lancet.* 2004 Sep 25–Oct 1;364(9440):1173–82. doi: 10.1016/S0140-6736(04)17107-9.
8. Leung AKC, Hon KL, Leong KF, Barankin B, Lam JM. Tinea capitis: an updated review. *Recent Pat Inflamm Allergy Drug Discov.* 2020;14(1):58–68.
9. Al Aboud AM, Crane JS. Tinea capitis. 2023 Aug 8. In: *StatPearls [Internet].* Treasure Island (FL): StatPearls Publishing; 2024 Jan–. PMID: 30725594.
10. Elghblawi E. Idiosyncratic findings in trichoscopy of tinea capitis: comma, zigzag hairs, corkscrew, and Morse code-like hair. *Int J Trichology.* 2016;8(4):180–3.
11. Dall'Oglio F, Nasca MR, Gerbino C, Micali G. An overview of the diagnosis and management of seborrheic dermatitis. *Clin Cosmet Investig Dermatol.* 2022 Aug 6;15:1537–48.
12. Bruni F, Alessandrini A, Starace M, Orlando G, Piraccini BM. Clinical and trichoscopic features in various forms of scalp psoriasis. *J Eur Acad Dermatol Venereol.* 2021 Sep;35(9):1830–7.
13. Starace M, Bruni F, Marcondes MT, Alessandrini A, Piraccini BM. The identification of trichoscopic features of allergic scalp contact dermatitis: a pilot-study of a single center. *Ital J Dermatol Venerol.* 2023 Aug;158(4):334–40.
14. Alessandrini A, Bruni F, Piraccini BM, Starace M. Common causes of hair loss – clinical manifestations, trichoscopy and therapy. *J Eur Acad Dermatol Venereol.* 2021 Mar;35(3):629–40.
15. Ekiz O, Sen BB, Rifaioğlu EN, Balta I. Trichoscopy in paediatric patients with tinea capitis: a useful method to differentiate from alopecia areata. *J Eur Acad Dermatol Venereol.* 2014 Sep;28(9):1255–8.
16. Melo DF, Lima CDS, Piraccini BM, Tosti A. Trichotillomania: what do we know so far? *Skin Appendage Disord.* 2022 Jan;8(1):1–7.

17. Żychowska M, Żychowska M. Dermoscopy of discoid lupus erythematosus – a systematic review of the literature. *Int J Dermatol.* 2021 Jul;60(7):818–28.

18. Vañó-Galván S, Molina-Ruiz AM, Fernández-Crehuet P, Rodrigues-Barata AR, Arias-Santiago S, Serrano-Falcón C, Martorell-Calatayud A, Barco D, Pérez B, Serrano S, Requena L, Grimalt R, Paoli J, Jaén P, Camacho FM. Folliculitis decalvans: a multicentre review of 82 patients. *J Eur Acad Dermatol Venereol.* 2015 Sep;29(9):1750–7.

19. Tangjaturonrusamee C, Piraccini BM, Vincenzi C, Starace M, Tosti A. Tinea capitis mimicking folliculitis decalvans. *Mycoses.* 2011 Jan;54(1):87–8. doi: 10.1111/j.1439-0507.2009.01761.x.

20. Lawson CN, Bakayoko A, Callender VD. Central centrifugal cicatricial alopecia: challenges and treatments. *Dermatol Clin.* 2021 Jul;39(3):389–405.

15

Trichoscopy of Tinea Capitis

Anna Waśkiel-Burnat, Marta Kurzeja, Agnieszka Michalczyk, and Lidia Rudnicka

15.1 Introduction

A mycological examination is considered as the gold standard diagnostic method in tinea capitis. Trichoscopy may be useful in making a correct diagnosis before culture results are available [1].

Trichoscopy, hair and scalp dermoscopy and videodermoscopy, is an easy-to-perform, non-invasive method helpful in diagnosing numerous hair and scalp disorders [2].

It was reported that trichoscopy is characterized by a higher sensitivity in diagnosing tinea capitis compared to direct examination (94% vs. 49.1%). Moreover, a high specificity (83%) of trichoscopy in diagnosis of tinea capitis was shown [3].

15.2 Trichoscopic Findings of Tinea Capitis

Trichoscopic features of tinea capitis are summarized in Table 15.1.

15.2.1 Comma Hairs

Comma hairs are short, C-shaped hairs (Figure 15.1). They are homogeneous in pigmentation and thickness [4]. Comma hairs result from subsequent cracking and bending of a hair shaft filled with hyphae [5].

TABLE 15.1

Trichoscopy of Tinea Capitis

Trichoscopic Findings in Tinea Capitis
Comma hairs
Corkscrew hairs
Morse code-like hairs
Zigzag hairs
Bent hairs
Block hairs
i-hairs
Black dots
Broken hairs
Scaling

DOI: 10.1201/9781003381648-17

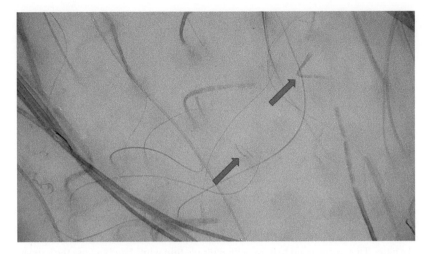

FIGURE 15.1
Comma hairs (short, C-shaped hairs) in a patient with tinea capitis.

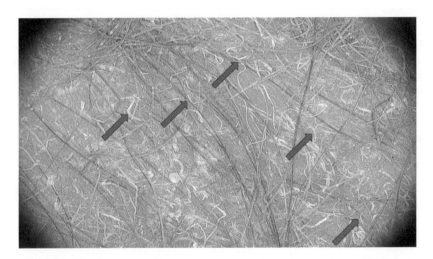

FIGURE 15.2
Corkscrew hairs in a patient with tinea capitis.

15.2.2 Corkscrew Hairs

Corkscrew hairs (Figure 15.2) represent multiple twisted and coiled hairs with corkscrew-like structure [4].

15.3 Morse Code-Like Hairs

Morse code-like hairs (Figure 15.3), also known as bar code-like hairs, correspond to hairs with multiple thin white bands across the hair shaft [4]. They are formed due to the accumulation of spores around the hair that cause a transverse perforation of the hair shaft [3].

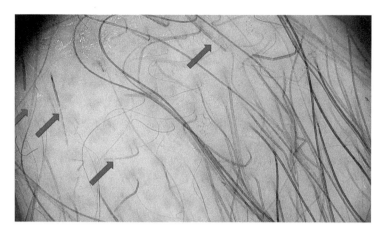

FIGURE 15.3
Morse code-like hairs. They correspond to hairs with multiple thin white bands across the hair shaft.

15.4 Zigzag Hairs

Zigzag hairs (Figure 15.4) are bent hairs with multiple sharp angles. They result from incomplete, transverse fractures along the hair shaft.

15.5 Bent Hairs

Bent hairs (Figure 15.5) are characterized by bending of the hair shaft [6]. They are normal long, homogeneous in thickness and pigmentation [7].

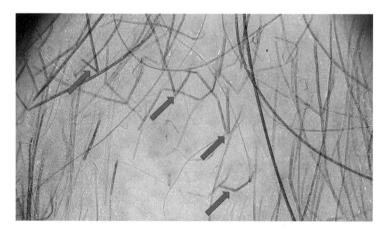

FIGURE 15.4
Zigzag hairs – bent hairs with multiple sharp angles.

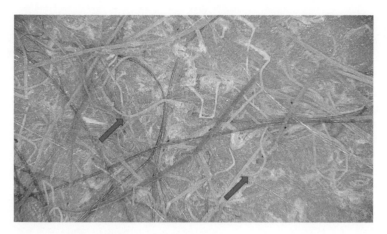

FIGURE 15.5
Bent hairs in a patient with tinea capitis.

15.6 Block Hairs and i-Hairs

Block hairs correspond to very short hairs with a transverse horizontal distal end. i-Hairs additionally have an accented dark distal end [8].

15.7 Other Trichoscopic Findings of Tinea Capitis

Other common, but not characteristic, trichoscopic findings of tinea capitis are broken hairs (Figure 15.6), black dots and scaling (Figure 15.7). In tinea capitis, both perifollicular and intrafollicular scaling is observed [2].

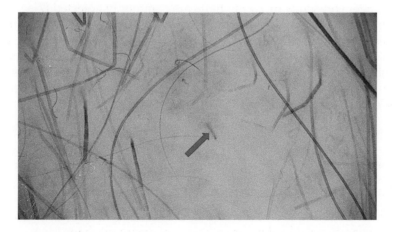

FIGURE 15.6
Broken hairs are commonly observed in patients with tinea capitis. However, they are not a characteristic finding.

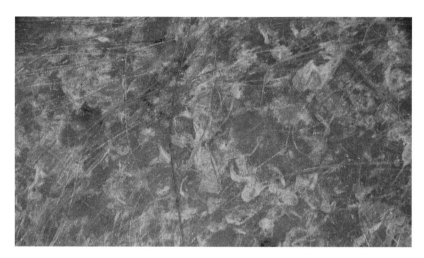

FIGURE 15.7
Scaling is a common feature of tinea capitis. It can be diffuse or perifollicular.

15.8 Trichoscopic Differences between *Microsporum* and *Trichophyton* Tinea Capitis

It was hypothesized that in endothrix-type fungal infection (particularly *Trichophyton*) the deformation of the hair shaft without an impairment of the colour is observed [7]. The hair shaft filled with hyphae breaks easily near the follicular ostia, thus a large number of short comma hairs and black dots are present on trichoscopy [9]. On the contrary, it was suggested that in ectothrix infection (particularly *Microsporum*) there is accumulation of spores around the hair shaft which causes transverse perforation of the hair shaft [7]. White, thin bands across the hair shaft which form Morse code-like appearance are observed. Transverse fractures of the hair shaft are presented farther from the follicular ostia. Thus, longer corkscrew or zigzag hairs are commonly detected [7].

Indeed, the systemic review and analysis from 2022 [2] on trichoscopic findings in tinea capitis showed that Morse code-like hairs, zigzag hairs, bent hairs and diffuse scaling were only present in *Microsporum* tinea capitis. On the contrary, corkscrew hairs were more commonly observed in *Trichophyton* compared to *Microsporum* tinea capitis [2]. Further studies are needed to confirm the usefulness of trichoscopy in differentiation between *Microsporum* and *Trichophyton* infection.

15.9 Trichoscopy in the Monitoring of Treatment Efficacy

Trichoscopy can also be used in the monitoring of treatment efficacy [2]. Effective therapy of tinea capitis is characterized by the disappearance of dystrophic hairs (such as short broken hairs, comma hairs, corkscrew hairs, black dots, i-hairs) 4–12 weeks after therapy initiation. Scaling tends to resolve more slowly and can be present in patients with negative mycological examination; thus, it should not be considered as a marker of therapy failure [10].

References

1. Aqil N, BayBay H, Moustaide K, Douhi Z, Elloudi S, Mernissi FZ. A prospective study of tinea capitis in children: making the diagnosis easier with a dermoscope. *J Med Case Rep.* 2018;12(1):383.
2. Waśkiel-Burnat A, Rakowska A, Sikora M, Ciechanowicz P, Olszewska M, Rudnicka L. Trichoscopy of tinea capitis: a systematic review. *Dermatol Ther (Heidelb)*. 2020;10(1):43–52.
3. Dhaille F, Dillies AS, Dessirier F, Reygagne P, Diouf M, Baltazard T, et al. A single typical trichoscopic feature is predictive of tinea capitis: a prospective multicentre study. *Br J Dermatol.* 2019;181(5):1046–51.
4. Rudnicka L, Rakowska A, Kerzeja M, Olszewska M. Hair shafts in trichoscopy: clues for diagnosis of hair and scalp diseases. *Dermatol Clin.* 2013;31(4):695–708, x.
5. Slowinska M, Rudnicka L, Schwartz RA, Kowalska-Oledzka E, Rakowska A, Sicinska J, et al. Comma hairs: a dermatoscopic marker for tinea capitis: a rapid diagnostic method. *J Am Acad Dermatol.* 2008;59(5 Suppl):S77–9.
6. Rudnicka L, Olszewska M, Rakowska A, Slowinska M. Trichoscopy update 2011. *J Dermatol Case Rep.* 2011;5(4):82–8.
7. Bourezane Y, Bourezane Y. Analysis of trichoscopic signs observed in 24 patients hpresenting tinea capitis: hypotheses based on physiopathology and proposed new classification. *Ann Dermatol Venereol.* 2017;144(8–9):490–6.
8. Rudnicka L Olszewska M, Rakowska A. *Atlas of trichoscopy.* Springer; 2012.
9. Schechtman RC, Silva ND, Quaresma MV, Bernardes Filho F, Buçard AM, Sodré CT. Dermatoscopic findings as a complementary tool in the differential diagnosis of the etiological agent of tinea capitis. *An Bras Dermatol.* 2015;90(3 Suppl 1):13–15.
10. Campos S, Brasileiro A, Galhardas C, Apetato M, Cabete J, Serrão V, et al. Follow-up of tinea capitis with trichoscopy: a prospective clinical study. *J Eur Acad Dermatol Venereol.* 2017;31(11):e478–80.

16

Mycological Examination of the Hair

Pauline Lecerf

The diagnosis of tinea capitis (TC) is based on clinical examination and laboratory tests. The former includes taking the patient's history (disease course, other affected individuals among the patient's social contacts, exposure to animals, trips abroad) and inspection (type of involvement, other clinical manifestations of dermatophytosis such as *tinea corporis* or onychomycosis) [1] (Table 16.1).

The Wood's lamp, an instrument with an ultraviolet light of 320–400 nm spectrum, has classically been used as a preliminary tool in the diagnosis of *tinea capitis*. It is particularly a useful diagnostic tool for diagnosing *tinea capitis* due to ectothrix *Microsporum species* (fluoresces a light, bright green), while *tinea capitis* caused by *Trichophyton* species does not fluoresce. *Trichophyton schoenleinii* fluoresces a blue/dull green fluorescence under the lamp (Figure 16.1a and b).

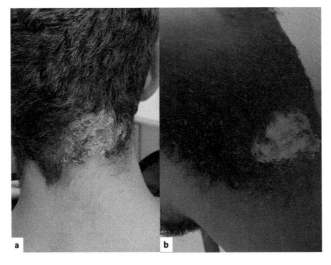

FIGURE 16.1
Microsporic *tinea capitis:* (a) clinical aspect; (b): Wood's lamp aspect.

DOI: 10.1201/9781003381648-18

TABLE 16.1

The Different Types of *Tinea Capitis*: Parasitism, Wood's Lamp Aspects, Clinical Manifestations and Responsible Agents

Type of Parasitism	Wood's Lamp	Pathogen	Ecological Niches	Clinical Pattern	Clinical Manifestations
Favic	+	*Trichophyton schoenleinii*	Anthropophilic	Favic	Thick yellow crusts "scutula", no broken hair to scarring alopecia in chronic infection
Endothrix	–	*Trichophyton tonsurans* *Trichophyton violaceum* *Trichophyton soudanense*		Trichophytic	Multiple irregular, erythematous scaling alopecic patches of 0.5–1 cm in diameter, broken hair at 1–2 mm form the scalp surface, obscured under layers of scales – "black dots" aspect
Endo-ectothrix microsporic	+	*Microsporum canis* *Microsporum audouinii* *Microsporum ferrugineum*	Zoophilic Anthropophilic	Microsporic	1–3 wide patches (2–6 cm in diameter) of broken hairs at 2–3 mm above the surface of the scalp
Endo-ectothrix microid	–	*Trichophyton mentagrophytes* *Trichophyton erinacei*	Zoophilic geophilic	Suppurativa (kerion)	Large, confluent, pus, painful, locoregional adenopathy scarring alopecia
Endo-ectothrix megaspore	–	*Trichophyton verrucosum* *Nannizzia gypsea*			

16.1 Sampling

In order to obtain valid test results, the sampling must be performed appropriately, preferably using sterile instruments. Suspicious lesions (if necessary, the site is determined by Wood's lamp examination or trichoscopy) should be disinfected with alcohol (70%), particularly if superinfection is suspected. In case of deep-seated inflammatory lesions, yellow crusts that may be present should be removed with tweezers.

A blunt instrument such as the back of a scalpel blade is useful for obtaining scales from the active edge of a suspected *tinea* infection. Using tweezers, hairs should be plucked from the periphery of the lesion, which can be done effortlessly (due to the inflammation). In lesions characterized by only minimal inflammation, scales and hairs should be collected using either the blunt end of a scalpel or by using the brush-culture or the swab method. The brush-culture can be directly inoculated onto the culture medium [1].

Swabs for mycology culture are useful to sample fungal kerions and pustular or macerated infections. The swab method may be performed with sterile cotton swabs, toothbrushes or cytobrushes (used for cervical swabs) [2,3]. The two-swab method is also suitable for use in the context of molecular pathogen identification. Brush or swab methods have the disadvantage of providing no material for direct microscopy. A retrospective study revealed the brush method to be statistically significantly superior to the scalpel method in terms of collecting material for pathogen detection; however, the highest sensitivity was achieved with a combination of both methods [1]. It is therefore recommended to use a combination of both techniques in the diagnostic workup. If only one method can be employed, the culture-brush method should be given preference [4].

The material collected should be transported in dark paper to the mycology laboratory for microscopy and culture. It is better to not use plastic containers, such as sterile specimen jars, because the scale sticks to the plastic (owing to static electricity).

16.2 Laboratory

16.2.1 Direct Microscopic Examination

Direct examination with potassium hydroxide (KOH) preparation and culture are the most commonly employed tests. KOH mount is a simple, rapid and inexpensive test that requires minimal infrastructure, though some amount of experience is necessary to interpret the smears accurately. Direct microscopy for hair is the same procedure as the one detailed in the chapter "Mycological Examination of the Nail". Well-prepared specimens that are only briefly incubated with KOH (otherwise there is too much damage to the hair structure) allow the distinction between ectothrix and endothrix infections. During the microscopic examination, the specimen is carefully observed under a microscope, employing a systematic approach that begins with low magnification and progressively increases as needed for detailed analysis. The objective is to identify various fungal elements within the sample. These microscopic characteristics play a crucial role in distinguishing different dermatophytes and determining the specific fungal species responsible for the infection:

- *Endothrix infections* (e.g. *Trichophyton tonsurans*):
  The fungal elements are primarily within the hair shaft. Arthrospores and hyphae may be visible inside the hair shaft, often causing it to break, leading to a "comma" or "black dot" appearance.

- *Ectothrix infections* (e.g. *Microsporum species*):
  The fungal elements surround the hair shaft. Hyphae and spores are seen on the external surface of the hair, forming a characteristic spore chain (Figure 16.2).

In addition to fungal elements, the presence of inflammatory cells like neutrophils or eosinophils may be noted, depending on the stage of the infection.

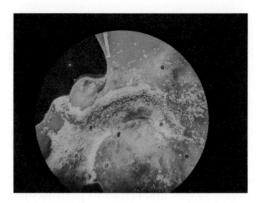

FIGURE 16.2
Direct microscopic examination of a hair in a microsporic *tinea capitis*.

16.2.2 Fungal Culture

Scales and hairs should be placed onto the agar, while hairs should be "planted" into the growth medium with their roots (Figure 16.3). The fungal culture derived from hair follows the same procedure as the one outlined in the chapter on the "mycological examination of nails". Dermatophytes typically exhibit growth within a timeframe of 2–6 weeks, a duration influenced by the specific species involved. This cultivation process serves as a meticulous means for accurately identifying the causative agent of the infection. However, it's essential to note that this method carries a 30% false-negative rate, emphasizing the importance of considering complementary diagnostic approaches for a comprehensive assessment.

16.2.3 Histological Examination of the Hair

In cases where pretreated patients yield negative results in mycological tests, a judicious approach involves the histological examination of biopsies, coupled with the application of fungal stains such as Periodic acid–Schiff (PAS) and Calcofluor white. Additionally, when necessary, polymerase chain reaction (PCR) may be employed for a more comprehensive evaluation. This is especially true for patients with deep dermatophytosis, as skin scrapings may contain only very few fungal elements in such cases. Saprophytic colonization of hair follicles by *Malassezia* spp. is an important differential diagnosis that should not be misinterpreted as TC [1].

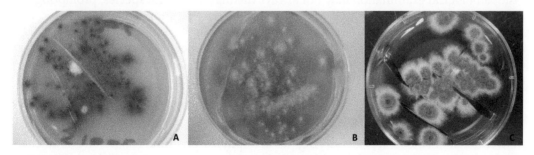

FIGURE 16.3
Fungal culture derived from hair in *tinea capitis*. Hair was planted in Sabouraud's medium with their roots.
(a): *Trichophyton tonsurans*; (b): *Microsporum audouinii*; (c) *Trichophyton soudanense*.

In cases of endothrix tinea capitis, the presence of spores and/or hyphae within the hair shaft is a common and distinctive feature. Ectothrix infections, such as *Microsporum canis*, involve fungi surrounding the hair shaft. Although there may be a superficial and/or deep perifollicular infiltration full of neutrophils, eosinophils and lymphocytes, the level of inflammation seen in histology varies greatly [5].

In *tinea capitis*, the infection starts from the perifollicular epidermis. The hyphae extend downwards from the follicle, invading the hair, first into the cuticle and then into the hair cortex. Dermatophytes causing endothrix infections exhibit round and box-like arthrospores, while those causing ectothrix infections form a sheath on the hair shaft surface. Perifollicular inflammation becomes apparent in advanced stages, with intense inflammation against foreign materials and degenerated follicle structures passing into the dermis. Dermal inflammation extends to subcutaneous and perivascular areas, characterized by a mixed dermal infiltrate of various immune cells. Additional findings are observed in kerion celsi and favus.

Histopathologically, **kerion celsi** is characterized by an inflammatory reaction with neutrophilic and/or granulomatous infiltrates, leading to fibrotic scarring. Severe inflammation in kerion can result in follicular destruction, causing granulomatous inflammation. Different histological patterns include suppurative folliculitis, suppurative folliculitis with suppurative dermatitis, suppurative folliculitis with suppurative and granulomatous dermatitis, and fibrosing dermatitis. Despite dramatic clinical signs, it may be challenging to locate infected follicles, requiring serial sections and fungal cultures for a definitive diagnosis [5,6].

Favus, caused by *Trichophyton schoenleinii*, involves the invasion of hair, creating air spaces without visible arthrospores and causing minor damage to hair shafts. Fungal elements are observed on the acanthotic epidermis, surrounding follicular ostia. The underlying dermis shows a mixed inflammatory infiltrate with giant cells and marked fibrosis, resembling folliculitis keloidalis [5].

The use of histopathology in diagnosing *tinea capitis* has two main disadvantages. Firstly, it is challenging to distinguish *tinea capitis* from other fungal infections (*Candida* sp., *Malassezia* sp., etc.). Secondly, fungal elements cannot be detected in all cases. Various special stains, such as PAS and Grocott methenamine silver (GMS), can aid in identifying fungal infections, but they have their limitations, including potential confusion between yeast and melanin granules and the need to differentiate hyphae from other structures. Fluorescence microscopy can help overcome some disadvantages of histopathological staining, as autofluorescence can be observed in sections stained with haematoxylin and eosin (H&E) and PAS. However, this method requires fluorescence microscopy [7]. Routine histopathological examination may not always distinguish fungal species, prompting the use of in situ hybridization with specific probes for detecting fungal nucleic acids.

In recent years, faster and less complex PCR methods have been utilized for detecting dermatophytes in histopathological sections, with higher sensitivity compared to traditional staining methods. Specifically, the sensitivity of detecting dermatophytes was reported to be 74% with PAS staining and 95% with ITS2 PCR [8].

16.2.4 Molecular Methods for Pathogen Identification

Conventional methods for identifying dermatophytes are time-consuming and challenging as they require specialized knowledge and are not always sufficiently discriminating to provide species-level identification. Molecular techniques such as PCR and matrix-assisted desorption/ionization time-of-flight mass spectrometry (MALDI-TOF MS) are increasingly used as more rapid, sensitive and accurate methods to identify dermatophyte species.

PCR-based methods, including conventional PCR, nested PCR and real-time PCR, offer swift and precise diagnosis, enabling accurate species-level identification of dermatophytes directly from clinical samples. The rDNA internal transcribed spacer (ITS) regions are commonly employed nucleotide sequences, along with other molecular markers such as partial ribosomal large subunit, ribosomal 60S protein, β-tubulin fragments and translation elongation factor [9]. Nested PCR, a post-PCR technique, involves a second amplification to enhance specificity and sensitivity by minimizing nonspecific binding of products from the initial PCR. Real-time PCR quantitatively estimates fungal load and helps differentiate infection from contamination based on threshold values. The closed tube system in real-time PCR minimizes contamination risks during the amplification and detection of pathogen DNA. Numerous commercial kits and in-house real-time PCR techniques have been developed to aid in the identification of dermatophytes. Studies indicate that real-time PCR significantly improves the detection rate of dermatophytes compared to traditional culture methods. Moreover, real-time PCR is effective in identifying co-infections (polyparasitism) in clinical samples [9,10].

PCR-based techniques are currently the only methods that allow for species identification from clinical material. Both in-house tests and commercially available test systems (kits) may be used for this purpose [1].

MALDI-TOF MS has become a powerful tool for dermatophyte identification alongside traditional morphological and DNA-based methods. It offers the advantages of rapid detection, high accuracy and ease of use compared to DNA-based techniques. A meta-analysis by Chen et al. revealed a high accuracy of MALDI-TOF MS in identifying dermatophytes, with a genus-level identification ratio of 0.96 and a species-level ratio of 0.91. Despite its effectiveness, MALDI-TOF MS hasn't been widely applied for dermatophyte detection from direct hair samples. Successful identification relies on a comprehensive database and an efficient protein extraction method. Challenges arise with moulds growing inside solid media, making hyphae collection difficult and often leading to low identification scores. A new culture medium, ID Fungi Plate (IDFP), has been developed to improve identification by facilitating clean harvests.

The IDFP, with a transparent membrane on the agar surface, enhances MALDI-TOF MS spectra generation for dermatophytes compared to traditional plates. However, it has a lower positive rate of fungal culture. While MALDI-TOF MS is effective, its widespread use is limited due to its high cost and the dependence on laboratory-established databases. In China, only a few mycologic laboratories can carry out this test. For competent laboratories, MALDI-TOF MS offers a rapid and highly accurate method for pathogen identification [9,11].

Flow cytometry is a technique used to analyse and quantify the physical and chemical characteristics of particles, usually cells, in a fluid as they pass through a laser beam.

Cells are labelled with fluorescent markers, and the emitted light is detected by photodetectors, providing information about cell size, granularity and the presence of specific surface markers. Flow cytometry is a powerful analytical technique used in various fields, including medical diagnostics, immunology and cell biology. Its application specifically in *tinea capitis* is relatively limited compared to other diagnostic methods. However, flow cytometry may have some potential applications in research or specific diagnostic scenarios related to *tinea capitis*.

References

1. Mayser P, Nenoff P, Reinel D, et al. S1 guidelines: tinea capitis. *JDDG J Dtsch Dermatol Ges.* 2020;18(2):161–79.
2. Bonifaz A, Isa-Isa R, Araiza J, et al. Cytobrush-culture method to diagnose tinea capitis. *Mycopathologia.* 2007;163(6):309–13.
3. Friedlander SF, Pickering B, Cunningham BB, Gibbs NF, Eichenfield LF. Use of the cotton swab method in diagnosing tinea capitis. *Pediatrics.* 1999;104(2 Pt 1):276–9.
4. Gupta AK, Friedlander SF, Simkovich AJ. Tinea capitis: an update. *Pediatr Dermatol.* 2022;39(2):167–72.
5. Elmas ÖF, Durdu M. Histopathology in the diagnosis of tinea capitis: when to do, how to interpret? *Mycopathologia.* 2023;188(5):545–52.
6. Arenas R, Toussaint S, Isa-Isa R. Kerion and dermatophytic granuloma. Mycological and histopathological findings in 19 children with inflammatory tinea capitis of the scalp. *Int J Dermatol.* 2006;45(3):215–19.
7. Estela Cubells JR, Victoria Martínez AM, Martínez Leboráns L, Alegre de Miquel V. Fluorescence microscopy as a diagnostic tool for dermatophytosis. *Am J Dermatopathol.* 2016;38(3):208–10.
8. Eckert JC, Ertas B, Falk TM, et al. Species identification of dermatophytes in paraffin-embedded biopsies with a new polymerase chain reaction assay targeting the internal transcribed spacer 2 region and comparison with histopathological features. *Br J Dermatol.* 2016;174(4):869–77.
9. Wei LW, Qiao JJ. Mini-review: The diagnostic methods of tinea capitis. *Mycopathologia.* 2023;188(5):563–19.
10. Verrier J, Monod M. Diagnosis of dermatophytosis using molecular biology. *Mycopathologia.* 2017;182(1–2):193–202.
11. Lecerf P, De Paepe R, Jazaeri Y, et al. Evaluation of a liquid media MALDI-TOF MS protocol for the identification of dermatophytes isolated from tinea capitis infections. *J Fungi Basel Switz.* 2022;8(12):1248.

17

Goals for the Treatment of Scalp Infection

Ditte Marie L. Saunte

The goals for the treatment of fungal scalp infections, tinea capitis, are to effectively eradicate the fungus causing the infection, relieve symptoms, promote healing of the affected scalp, prevent complications and prevent societal spread of the infection.

17.1 Eradicating the Fungus and Preventing Complications

Species and genus-directed antifungal therapy is initiated to stop the disease progression, eradicate the fungus and cure the patient. This means that an essential prerequisite for starting treatment is identification of the causative organism as this will guide the selection of the appropriate antifungal. Please see the chapter of Tinea capitis treatment for information on antifungal therapy for the scalp.

The treatment is also facilitated to initiate the healing process. The clinical manifestations of scalp infection may differ between the individual patients according to their immune response and the dermatophyte species involved. Some patients present with severely painful inflammation (kerion celsi) which can destroy hair follicles and lead to permanent scarring in up to 27.5% of the patients (Figure 17.1) [1]. The clinical presentation is sometimes confused with bacterial infection and surgical attempts to make an incision are without effect and may even cause scarring.

Kerion celsi is mainly caused by zoophilic infections transmitted from an animal to a human, causing a pronounced inflammation in contrast to anthropophilic infections that

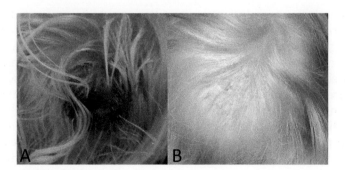

FIGURE 17.1
Treatment evaluation of a patient with kerion caused by *Trichophyton mentagrophytes*. (a) Kerion. (b) Follow-up after 4 months of terbinafine treatment. Negative direct microscopy and culture. Sequelae scaling and alopecia.

DOI: 10.1201/9781003381648-19

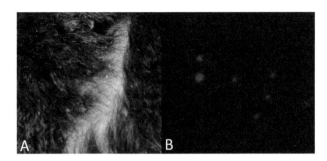

FIGURE 17.2
Treatment evaluation of patient with tinea capitis caused by *Trichophyton violaceum*. (a) Discrete dandruff, no broken hairs or alopecia. (b) Different sizes of conidia visualized by direct microscopy with fluorescent microscope 40× magnification using 10% potassium hydroxide (KOH) with Blankophor.

predominantly are non-inflammatory and tends to be more persistent (Figure 17.2) [1,2]. Scarring is rare in endothrix infections, but may occur after severe inflammation [2,3]. It is therefore important to reduce the inflammation to prevent scarring, and corticosteroids have historically been used as an adjunct therapy in tinea capitis, which at least in theory should also reduce the risk of scarring [4]. It is, however, not recommended anymore as studies have shown that they do not reduce the time to clinical and mycological cure as compared to antifungals alone [3–6].

17.2 Clinical and Mycological Treatment Evaluation

17.2.1 Clinical Treatment Evaluation

Clinical cure with hair regrowth and no signs of infection such as broken hairs, skin scales, crusts or pus is important, but the primary treatment goal is eradication of the fungus, mycological cure. Mycological cure may be difficult to evaluate clinically, especially in patients in whom haircare includes the use of oil products. It is therefore important to collect scalp specimens to perform a mycological evaluation.

17.2.2 Specimen Collection

Collection of material for mycological examination should be performed thoroughly, e.g. by using a hairbrush, tooth brush, a comb to massage the scalp, thus loosening skin scales and weakly attached hairs [7]. Wood's lamp examination (UV lamp emitting ultraviolet radiation of 365 nm) is helpful to determine the treatment response in patients with a *Microsporum* infection (or *Trichophyton schoenleinii* which is rare) as these dermatophytes fluoresce blue-green when exposure by light [3,8]. It is important to note that the optimal areas for sampling are those where there is hair fluorescence or clinical signs of infection such as broken hairs (black dots), skin scales, crusting or pustules. Sometimes, though rarely, the scalp presents as clinically cured, but retains positive fluorescence and may grow a dermatophyte. This underlines the utility of using the Wood's lamp.

Trichoscopy is also a useful non-invasive bedside tool, which is helpful for treatment control and to determine the most optimal area for specimen collection [9].

It is important to note that neither Wood's light nor trichoscopy is able to determine the viability of the fungus involved.

17.2.3 Mycological Examination

Mycological eradication is the most important treatment goal. A positive direct micros-copy with detection of fungal elements is a sign of infection but does not determine if the fungus is living [10]. Molecular-based methods such as, e.g. polymerase chain reac-tion (PCR) and matrix-assisted laser desorption ionization–time of flight (MALDI-TOF) are able to diagnose dermatophytes to species level but yet, again, are not able to confirm fun-gal viability, but developments may allow them to do so in the future. The fungal growth on a suitable media (culture) is currently the only method to assess the fungal viability [10]. Another advantage of the fungal culture is that it can be extended to antifungal sus-ceptibility testing [10].

Patients with negative mycology and clinical normalization are considered cured, whereas patients with scars and negative mycological examination are considered cured but with sequelae.

Patients that are clinically cured, but have a positive mycological examination are con-sidered asymptomatic carriers and may serve as a fungal reservoir and therefore a source of disease transmission.

17.3 Preventing Societal Spread

It is important to prevent societal spread of tinea capitis. The risk of wider spread is higher if the infection is caused by an anthropophilic species as they are transmitted between humans and mostly present clinically with discrete signs of infection. Family members and close contacts to the index child should be screened for infection or asymptomatic carriage. Species-directed treatment should be initiated according to current guidelines, and if antifungal resistance is suspected antifungal susceptibility testing should be per-formed. It is important to explain that the patient should follow the plan as prescribed by a healthcare professional and to complete the full course of medication, even if symptoms improve. Fungal infections can be stubborn, and premature discontinuation of treatment may lead to a recurrence of the infection. Regular follow-up visits with the healthcare provider are essential to monitor progress and ensure complete resolution of the infection. The family should be instructed to perform a limited number of hygiene measures such as disinfection of fomites. Please see Chapter 18 for more details.

References

1. Friedland R, Sabbah F, Reiss-Huss S, et al. Epidemiologic features and risk of scarring in pedi-atric patients with kerion celsi. *Pediatr Dermatol*. 2022 Mar 1;39(2):215–9.
2. Hay RJ. Tinea capitis: current status. *Mycopathologia*. 2017;182(1–2):87–93.
3. Fuller LCC, Barton RCC, Mohd Mustapa MFF, et al. British Association of Dermatologists' guidelines for the management of tinea capitis 2014. *Br J Dermatol*. 2014;171(3):454–63.
4. Hussain I, Muzaffar F, Rashid T, et al. A randomized, comparative trial of treatment of kerion celsi with griseofulvin plus oral prednisolone vs. griseofulvin alone. *Med Mycol*. 1999;37(2):97–9.
5. Proudfoot LE, Higgins EM, Morris-Jones R. A retrospective study of the management of pedi-atric kerion in Trichophyton tonsurans infection. *Pediatr Dermatol*. 2011;28(6):655–7.

6. Honig PJ. Tinea capitis: recommendations for school attendance. *Pediatr Infect Dis J.* 1999;18(2):211–14.

7. Akbaba M, Ilkit M, Sutoluk Z, et al. Comparison of hairbrush, toothbrush and cotton swab methods for diagnosing asymptomatic dermatophyte scalp carriage. *J Eur Acad Dermatol Venereol.* 2008;22(3):356–62.

8. Wigger-Alberti W, Elsner P. Fluorescence with Wood's light. Current applications in dermatologic diagnosis, therapy follow-up and prevention. *Hautarzt.* 1997;48(8):523–7.

9. Wahbah HR, Atallah RB, Eldahshan RM, et al. A prospective clinical and trichoscopic study of tinea capitis in children during treatment. *Dermatol Ther.* 2022;35(7):e15582.

10. Saunte DML, Piraccini BM, Sergeev AY, et al. A survey among dermatologists: diagnostics of superficial fungal infections – what is used and what is needed to initiate therapy and assess efficacy? *J Eur Acad Dermatology Venereol.* 2018;33(2):421–7.

18

Treatment of Tinea Capitis

Roderick Hay

18.1 Introduction

Tinea capitis is a treatable infection that responds to oral antifungals, although in many resource-poor areas the drugs that are effective are unaffordable. This means that in many regions endemic for scalp ringworm there are large numbers of untreated children. Nonetheless there are certain principles that underlie planning the treatment of tinea capitis; these involve: (1) the treatment of the individual patient after confirming the diagnosis; (2) screening human and animal contacts to prevent further infection from the same source; and (3) prevention of spread of the infection to others in the community [1]. Successful treatment requires identification of the causative dermatophyte as this provides the best guide to choose the most suitable therapy. Where this is not possible, knowing the commonest causes of scalp infection in the area provides a pointer to the most likely suitable treatment options. In addition, there should be a clinical assessment of the infection including whether or not it is inflammatory, for instance, a kerion, or whether it has spread to other sites, e.g. face or body, followed by the initiation of the correct therapy. Standard diagnostic tools involve direct microscopy, culture or use of a molecular diagnostic tool such as polymerase chain reaction (PCR) or matrix-assisted laser desorption ionization–time of flight (MALDI-ToF) as discussed in Chapter 16.

Screening contacts involves careful examination of siblings and other members of the household to check whether they have concurrent infection. With anthropophilic infections, in apparently asymptomatic contacts, cultures of scalp brushes to establish the presence of carriage or infection are important. But if a zoophilic infection is suspected, animal contacts should be screened where possible for infection by a veterinarian. Laboratory-confirmed contacts, whether carriers or infected cases, should be treated (see below). In areas where access to diagnostic facilities is limited, it is reasonable to treat the child's household members as potential carriers with topical therapy (see below).

18.2 Treatment Options

18.2.1 Topical Antifungals

Topical antifungals are generally ineffective in the treatment of tinea capitis as opposed to asymptomatic carriers. There are no published studies about the penetration of topically applied agents applied to hair, and no antifungal formulations have been specifically

DOI: 10.1201/9781003381648-20

designed to provide high hair shaft drug concentrations. So, it is unlikely that any topically applied medication can produce growth inhibition of fungi in infected hairs or achieve levels associated with fungicidal activity.

18.2.1.1 As Primary Therapy

Furthermore, there have been few clinical trials that have investigated the efficacy of topical treatments in tinea capitis. However, one such study compared topical miconazole with Whitfield's ointment in a cohort of children with tinea capitis in Zimbabwe. This showed that patients receiving topical treatment had some limited clinical improvement and, in some children, negative cultures were obtained during therapy. But these numbers were not as high as those expected following treatment with oral antifungals (see below) and the patients achieving clinical or mycological cure with topical antifungals relapsed subsequently [2].

18.2.1.2 As Adjunctive Therapy

Topical antifungals are, however, often used as adjuncts to oral therapy to reduce the frequency of positive cultures from hair during the early stages of therapy and on the premise that they will reduce the risk of dissemination to other children through contact with infected hairs on clothing or fomites [3]. The antifungals used for this purpose have mainly been antifungals in shampoo formulations such as selenium sulphide and ketoconazole. Although other shampoos, such as those containing piroctone, potentially have antifungal activity, their role in reducing spread has not been explored. Treatment of carriers will be discussed later.

18.2.2 Oral Antifungal Treatments

Effective treatment of tinea capitis depends on the use of oral antifungal therapy.

18.2.2.1 Griseofulvin

The first effective treatment to be used for tinea capitis was griseofulvin. This drug is fungistatic in vitro against the dermatophytes that cause tinea capitis, and its mode of action is thought to be through the inhibition of the formation of intracellular microtubules in hyphae. Griseofulvin was widely used in the 1960s and 1970s to eliminate endemic tinea capitis in Europe and the USA. It is usually given in a dose of 10–15 mg/kg daily, for 6–8 weeks [3,4]. As griseofulvin was one of the earliest antifungal drugs to be introduced for human use there are few comparative clinical trials against placebo, although comparative studies against other antifungals were carried out later after griseofulvin's approval for this indication. For most organisms that cause tinea capitis, griseofulvin is clinically and mycologically effective. Patients with certain infections such as those caused by *Trichophyton tonsurans* require longer courses of treatment, e.g. 12 weeks and even so may fail to respond [5]. So, a higher dose of griseofulvin of 20 mg/kg/day has been recommended for *T. tonsurans* infections. Comparative treatment studies with griseofulvin are discussed later.

When griseofulvin was first introduced, it was recognized that it could provide an effective treatment for mass administration in areas where prevalence rates of tinea capitis in children were high. In response to this perceived need, higher doses of griseofulvin given as single treatments were found to be effective as part of a mass drug administration (MDA) approach for community-based treatments against certain endothrix infections, e.g. *Trichophyton violaceum* [6,7]. Dosage regimens varied, but 1 G given as a single dose or 500 mg as a stat dose followed by a repeat dose after 2 weeks were two such regimens employed to reduce the frequency of infection among children in communities. Single-dose treatments could also be given as supervised therapy. However, these dosage regimens were never widely used either for treating individuals or communities and they are not currently recommended for routine individual use.

The availability of different formulations of griseofulvin is also very variable from country to country. In some there are both tablet and oral suspension (ultra-microsize) formulations of griseofulvin, the latter being particularly helpful for younger children. However, in some countries, the liquid paediatric formulation of griseofulvin is difficult to obtain. Alternative formulations can be imported, or some local pharmacies have tried to address the problem by suspending crushed tablets of griseofulvin in a liquid base, although there is no published assessment of this approach to therapy.

Clinical trials comparing terbinafine with griseofulvin show similar efficacy in *Microsporum* and *Trichophyton* infections, but responses for *Trichophyton* species appear to be faster with the former [8,9] (see below). Griseofulvin performs well in *Microsporum* infections and in some cases appears more effective than alternative antifungals.

18.2.2.2 Terbinafine

Terbinafine is an allylamine drug with broad-spectrum in vitro antifungal activity and this includes those dermatophytes that cause tinea capitis. For scalp infections, terbinafine is available as a 250 mg tablet. In some countries, a paediatric tablet of 125 mg is available and in others terbinafine granules which are coated to disguise their taste have been licensed. The normal daily dose is 250 mg for adults. In children, the treatment regimen is based on weight: <20 kg: 62.5 mg/day, 20–40 kg: 125 mg/day and >40 kg: 250 mg/day. Although terbinafine is effective against a range of fungi that cause tinea capitis, the efficacy varies between different species; there are a number of studies comparing terbinafine with griseofulvin [8–11]. The recommended treatment length for most infections is usually 4 weeks.

Studies have shown that in infections caused by *T. tonsurans*, 4 weeks of treatment is required although shorter periods are sometimes effective. Some organisms appear to respond quicker. For instance, in a study of *T. violaceum* infection, there was no difference in the mycological cure rates at follow-up when 1 week of treatment was compared with 2 or 4 weeks of therapy [12]. A meta-analysis of studies comparing terbinafine with griseofulvin has also shown that terbinafine was as effective at treatment durations of up to 2–4 weeks for *Trichophyton* infections compared with griseofulvin for 6–8 weeks [9]. However, the responses of *Microsporum* species to this drug were slower than those of *Trichophyton*, and in some patients, there appears to be no response [13–15]. One way around this issue is to use higher doses of terbinafine, and for *Microsporum* infections, double the normal daily dose is therefore advised. Unfortunately, the choice of drug cannot be guided by in vitro sensitivity treating as isolates of *Microsporum* are not significantly less sensitive to terbinafine in vitro than those of *Trichophyton* [16]. So any differences are probably determined by whether the infecting dermatophyte is located around (ectothrix) or within the hair shaft (endothrix). Ectothrix infections generally respond less well to terbinafine. There is a recently reported association between treatment failure in *T. tonsurans* infection and the presence of co-existent tinea corporis [17]. Using terbinafine in granule form produces similar results. In other words, it is more effective in *Trichophyton* infections but not in *Microsporum* infections. So, changing the formulation does not appear to affect the clinical responses in any significant way [18].

As stated previously, in some countries, a paediatric terbinafine tablet of 125 mg or granules are available. An unsatisfactory option, for smaller children, is to break the 250 mg tablets, which may be scored (depending on source). There are generic forms of terbinafine available in some countries.

18.2.2.3 Itraconazole

Itraconazole is an orally active triazole antifungal which shows fungistatic activity in vitro against the main causes of tinea capitis. Itraconazole comes in three main formulations: a capsule containing pelleted itraconazole (Sporanox), an oral solution containing itraconazole in cyclodextrin and a newer solid formulation with better absorption (Subacap or Lozanoc). The latter is licensed in some countries in Europe, in Australia and South America for the treatment of dermatophyte infections but it has not been tested specifically for tinea capitis. There are also generic forms of itraconazole available in some countries.

For the treatment of tinea capitis, itraconazole is generally given in doses of 3–5 mg/kg daily. The doses used for this infection have varied between 3 and 5 mg/kg daily for periods of between 4 and 6 weeks [19–21]. Efficacy rates have varied from over 80% to 40%. As an alternative regimen using a pulsed approach to treatment, i.e. higher dose given at longer intervals, has been adopted by some [22]. There is no evidence that *Microsporum* and *Trichophyton* species causing tinea capitis differ in their responses to itraconazole. A pulsed regimen using intermittent treatment with 5 mg/kg/day for 1 week every 3 weeks has been evaluated in a small number of children. Usually two to three pulses were found to be effective for most scalp infections [22].

However, the pelleted capsule formulation is difficult to use in children on a dose per weight basis as it involves opening and dividing the contents of capsules. The oral solution is more easily adapted for paediatric use but its taste is bitter. This can be improved by mixing with a fruit juice, although this has only been studied in children using the medication in the presence of malignant disease rather than tinea capitis [23].

18.2.2.4 Fluconazole

Fluconazole is an orally active triazole antifungal, and there are both capsule and liquid formulations. The drug is active in vitro against a range of fungi including those dermatophytes that cause tinea capitis. The doses that have been used in tinea capitis have ranged from 1.5 to 6 mg/kg daily or as an intermittent regimen such as and up to 8 mg/kg weekly [24–26]. Fluconazole appears to be equally effective against a range of different organisms in tinea capitis including both *Trichophyton* and *Microsporum* species. It also appears to be as effective as griseofulvin [27,28]. The oral solution may be particularly helpful in young children.

18.2.2.4.1 Other Azoles

Other azoles in current usage such as posaconazole, voriconazole, isavuconazole have not been used in tinea capitis, although they are active in vitro against most dermatophytes that cause tinea capitis [20,29,30,31].

18.2.2.4.1.1 Treatment Guidelines The generally recommended treatment for tinea capitis due to Trichophyton species is terbinafine which is given for a 1-month period as the initial treatment of choice. For Microsporum infections, there remains a choice which is largely determined by drug availability and cost. Often the first choice is griseofulvin for 6–8 weeks; itraconazole or terbinafine (at double normal dose) are alternatives, and these are also given for 6–8 weeks. Often children are also treated with a topical agent to reduce the risk of spread in the early phase of oral treatment. Ketoconazole shampoo, twice or three times weekly for the first 2 weeks of oral therapy, is the most popular. National guidelines provide more detailed recommendations along these lines, e.g. British Association of Dermatologists [32] or the European Society for Paediatric Dermatology [33].

18.2.2.4.1.2 Treatment of Carriers Topically applied ketoconazole and selenium sulphide in shampoos reduce the frequency of positive cultures from both infected children and those carrying the organism without clinical evidence of infection [34–36]. Topical antifungals are recommended for carriers defined as asymptomatic children with positive brush cultures. If scalp brushes produce very heavy growth of fungus, it is likely that the children have a true but asymptomatic infection, and these should be treated as infected patients by using the appropriate oral antifungal. There is some concern that T. tonsurans detected by scalp brush, but not by direct microscopy, may reflect a true infection rather than carriage in some cases. Current advice is that wherever possible if T. tonsurans is identified by culture or molecular methods but not seen on microscopy children should be re-examined to check whether there is any clinical evidence to suggest hair shaft infection and then treated with oral therapy if there is proven infection.

18.2.2.4.2 Schools

While infected children pose a potential infectious risk to those who are not infected, the method by which the organisms spread from head to head is not known, e.g. aerosol and direct contact. Exclusion of infected children from school is not recommended in most countries.

Recent work suggests that treating whole classes, where there is a risk of infection, with ketoconazole shampoo to prevent infection is not effective [37].

18.2.2.4.2.1 Kerion In kerions the same treatment regimens as those used for children with other forms of tinea capitis are used. But it may be necessary to continue antifungal therapy for longer periods, e.g. 12–16 weeks. Some clinical trials have tried to address the use of systemic corticosteroids in kerions, and advice is based on anecdotal experience. The concurrent use of oral or topical corticosteroids has been recommended by some dermatologists – and not by others. The rational for their use is that they will reduce the intense inflammatory reaction that occurs with kerions. However, one trial which examined the value of oral corticosteroids found that their addition to the oral antifungal regimen made no difference to clinical and mycological response rates [38].

However, one practical approach to the treatment of kerions is that the removal of surface crusts is often helpful as it relieves itching and secondary infection. As it can be painful the procedure is best carried out after soaking the crusts with lukewarm water or saline applied topically in the form of moistened dressings. The softened crusts can then be gently teased away. Secondary bacterial infection, usually due to *Staphylococcus aureus*, should be treated with antibiotics such as flucloxacillin; however, pustules that may be seen in the lesions of kerion are more often a response to the fungus rather than bacterial infection. The application of an antifungal cream with anti-Gram-positive bacterial activity such as miconazole, clotrimazole or econazole may also allow the scalp to heal and prevent formation of new crusts.

References

1. Fuller LC, Child FJ, Midgley G, Higgins EM. Diagnosis and management of scalp ringworm. *BMJ* 2003;326:539–41.
2. Wright S, Robertson VJ. An institutional survey of tinea capitis in Harare, Zimbabwe and a trial of miconazole cream versus Whitfield's ointment in its treatment. *Clin Exp Dermatol.* 1986;11:371–7.
3. Michaels BD, Del Rosso JQ. Tinea capitis in infants: recognition, evaluation, and management suggestions. *J Clin Aesthet Dermatol.* 2012;5:49–59.
4. Stritzler C, Rein RL, Ulku K. Tinea capitis treated with griseofulvin: evaluation of dosage schedules and some immunological studies. *Arch Dermatol.* 1962;85(6):743–5.
5. Abdel-Rahman SM, Nahata MC, Powell DA. Response to initial griseofulvin therapy in pediatric patients with tinea capitis. *Ann Pharmacother.* 1997 Apr;31(4):406–10.
6. Beghin D, Vanbreuseghem R. Traitment des dermatophyties du cuir chevelu par une dose unique de griseofulvine; essai d'une dose reduite. *Ann Soc Belg Med Trop.* 1974;54:477–81.
7. Friedman L, Derbes VJ, Tromovitch TA. Single dose therapy of tinea capitis. *Arch Dermatol.* 1960;82(3):415–8.
8. Caceres-Rios H, Rueda M, Ballona R, Bustamante B. Comparison of terbinafine and griseofulvin in the treatment of tinea capitis. *J Am Acad Dermatol.* 2000;42:80–4.
9. Gupta AK, Drummond-Main C. Meta-analysis of randomized, controlled trials comparing particular doses of griseofulvin and terbinafine for the treatment of tinea capitis. *Pediatr Dermatol.* 2013;30:1–6.
10. Fuller LC, Smith CH, Cerio R et al., A randomized comparison of 4 weeks of terbinafine vs. 8 weeks of griseofulvin for the treatment of tinea capitis, *Br J Dermatol* 2001;144/2:321–7.
11. Khan SU, Khan AR, Wazir SM. Efficacy of terbinafine vs. griseofulvin in tinea capitis in the Northern areas of Pakis. *J Pak Assoc Dermatol.* 2016 Dec 22 [cited 2023 Oct 9];21(4):281–4.
12. Haroon TS, Hussain I, Aman S. A randomised double-blind comparative study of terbinafine for 1, 2 and 4 weeks in tinea capitis. *Br J Dermatol.* 1996;135:86–8.
13. Kullavanijaya P, Reangchainam S, Ungpakorn R. Randomized single-blind study of efficacy and tolerability of terbinafine in the treatment of tinea capitis. *J Am Acad Dermatol.* 1997;37:272–3.
14. Dragos V, Lunder M. Lack of efficacy of 6 week treatment with oral terbinafine for tinea capitis due to *Microsporum canis* in children. *Pediatr Dermatol.* 1997;14:46–8.
15. Devliotou-Panagiotidou D, Koussidou-Eremondi TH. Efficacy and tolerability of 8 weeks' treatment with terbinafine in children with tinea capitis caused by *Microsporum canis*: a comparison of three doses. *J Eur Acad Dermatol Venereol.* 2004;18:155–9.
16. Mock M, Monod M, Baudraz-Rosselet F, Panizzon RG. Tinea capitis, dermatophytes: susceptibility to antifungal drugs tested in vitro and in vivo. *Dermatology.* 1998;197:361–7.
17. Galili, E, Goldsmith, T, Khanimov, I, et al. Tinea capitis caused by *Trichophyton tonsurans* among adults: clinical characteristics and treatment response. *Mycoses.* 2023;66:144–9. doi: 10.1111/myc.13536n
18. Elewski BE, Cáceres HW, DeLeon L, et al. Terbinafine hydrochloride oral granules versus oral griseofulvin suspension in children with tinea capitis: results of two randomized, investigator-blinded, multicenter, international, controlled trials. *J Am Acad Dermatol.* 2008 Jul;59(1):41–54.
19. Lopez Gomez S, Del Palacio A, Van Cutsem J, et al. Itraconazole versus griseofulvin in the treatment of tinea capitis. A double blind randomised study in children. *Int J Dermatol.* 1994;33:743–7.
20. Abdel-Rahman SM, Powell DA, Nahata MC. Efficacy of itraconazole in children with *Trichophyton tonsurans* with tinea capitis. *J Am Acad Dermatol.* 1998;38:443–6.
21. Ginter-Hanselmayer G, Smolle J, Gupta A. Itraconazole in the treatment of tinea capitis caused by Microsporum canis: experience in a large cohort. *Pediatr Dermatol.* 2004;21:499–502.

22. Gupta AK, Alexis ME, Raboobee N. Itraconazole pulse therapy is effective in the treatment of tinea capitis in children: an open multicentre study. *Br J Dermatol.* 1997;137:251–4.
23. Adachi Y, Sumikuma T, Kagami R, et al. Improvement of patient adherence by mixing oral itraconazole solution with a beverage (orange juice). *Rinsho Ketsueki.* 2010 May;51(5):315–19.
24. Solomon BA, Collins R, Sharma R, et al. Fluconazole for the treatment of tinea capitis in children. *J Am Acad Dermatol.* 1997;37:274–5.
25. Mercurio MG, Silverman RA, Elewski BE. Tinea capitis: fluconazole in *Trichophyton tonsurans* infections. *Pediatr Dermatol.* 1998;37:274–5.
26. Gupta AK, Adam P, Hofstader Sl et al. Intermittent short duration therapy with fluconazole is effective for tinea capitis. *Br J Dermatol.* 1999;141:304–6.
27. Dastghaib L, Azizzadeh M, Jafari P. Therapeutic options for the treatment of tinea capitis: griseofulvin versus fluconazole. *J Dermatol Treat.* 2005;16:43–6.
28. Shemer A, Plotnik IB, Davidovici B, et al. Treatment of tinea capitis - griseofulvin versus fluconazole – a comparative study. *J Dtsch Dermatol Ges.* 2013;11:737–42.
29. Ghannoum M, Isham N, Sheehan D Voriconazole susceptibilities of dermatophyte isolates obtained from a worldwide tinea capitis clinical trial *J Clin Microbiol.* 2006;44:2579–80.
30. Barchiesi F, Arzeni D, Camiletti V, et al. In vitro activity of posaconazole against clinical isolates of dermatophytes. *J Clin Microbiol.* 2001 Nov;39(11):4208–9.
31. Badiee, P., Shokohi, T., Hashemi, J. et al. Comparison of in vitro activities of newer triazoles and classic antifungal agents against dermatophyte species isolated from Iranian university hospitals: a multi-central study. *Ann Clin Microbiol Antimicrob.* 2023;22:15.
32. Fuller LC, Barton RC, Mohd Mustapa MF, et al. British Association of Dermatologists' guidelines for the management of tinea capitis 2014. *Br J Dermatol.* 2014 Sep;171(3):454–63.
33. Kakourou T, Uksal U; European society for pediatric dermatology. Guidelines for the management of tinea capitis in children. *Pediatr Dermatol.* 2010;27(3):226–8.
34. McGinley KJ, Leyden JJ. Antifungal activity of dermatological shampoos. *Arch Dermatol Res.* 1982;272:339–42.
35. Allen HB, Honig PJ, Leyden JJ, McGinley KJ. Selenium sulfide: adjunctive therapy for tinea capitis. *Pediatrics.* 1982;69:81–3.
36. Greer DL. Successful treatment of tinea capitis with 2% ketoconazole shampoo. *Int J Dermatol.* 2000;39:302–4.
37. Bookstaver PB, Watson HJ, Winters SD, et al. Prophylactic ketoconazole shampoo for tinea capitis in a high-risk pediatric population. *J Pediatr Pharmacol Ther.* 2011;16:199–203.
38. Hussain I, Muzaffar F, Rashid T, Ahmad TJ, Jahangir M, Haroon TS. A randomized, comparative trial of treatment of kerion celsi with griseofulvin plus oral prednisolone vs. griseofulvin alone. *Med Mycol.* 1999;37:97–9.

19

Preventive Measures

Eduardo Corona-Rodarte, Luis Enrique Cano-Aguilar,
Roberto Arenas, and Daniel Asz-Sigall

19.1 Introduction

In the extensive field of dermatology, few conditions exemplify the persistent challenge posed by fungal infections as effectively as tinea capitis. This common, yet often perplexing condition, extends its influence beyond the boundaries of mere superficiality, deeply impacting personal well-being, social interactions and even livelihoods. The quest for effective preventive measures in combating these fungal challenges has spurred a convergence of knowledge, bridging the gap between human and veterinary approaches. A comprehensive understanding of the underlying factors and therapeutic strategies is crucial for effective management.

The significance of preventive measures in managing tinea capitis cannot be overstated. These measures offer a proactive approach that not only reduces the burden on affected individuals but also contributes to the broader efforts in healthcare. Preventive strategies encompass a spectrum of interventions, ranging from personal hygiene practices to public health campaigns. They target not only the infected individuals but also the environmental reservoirs of these fungi, thus addressing both transmission and persistence. Furthermore, achieving optimal cure rates hinges on a few key practices. This becomes remarkably important when dealing with longer treatment regimens. Ensuring strict adherence to the prescribed treatment plan is paramount. Taking medications exactly as directed by the healthcare provider plays a pivotal role in enhancing therapeutic outcomes. For instance, in the case of itraconazole, consuming it with food as indicated can significantly enhance its effectiveness. These conscientious steps not only contribute to maximizing cure rates but also exemplify the collaborative partnership between patients and healthcare professionals in the pursuit of successful management.

19.1.1 Tinea Capitis: A Comprehensive Perspective

Tinea capitis is a prevalent scalp hair infection primarily affecting children, resulting from dermatophytes. This condition demands not only clinical expertise but also a profound understanding of preventive measures that extend beyond individual cases.

Anthropophilic dermatophytes can spread through direct contact between humans or indirectly via items like hair care tools and toys. The prevailing mode is thought to be the indirect route, as dermatophytes primarily disseminate through the shedding of infected skin cells and hair. The shared factor contributing to transmission is intimate physical proximity; nevertheless, it is not advised to exclude or isolate patients in schools or daycare

DOI: 10.1201/9781003381648-21

facilities to effectively prevent tinea capitis [1]. Medical professionals should emphasize avoiding the sharing of personal items like hats, hairbrushes, combs, pillows and helmets, as this minimizes its potential for fungal transmission. Ensuring optimal scalp hygiene for young patients through cleanliness and dryness is crucial. Caution is advised when considering environments with a high risk of infection acquisition. Frequently laundering pillows, sheets and bedding helps eliminate potential sources of contamination, creating a hygienic sleeping environment. Additionally, advocating for meticulous hand hygiene practices, especially after pet interactions, mitigates the risk of tinea capitis transmission from animals to individuals. After successful treatment, continuing the application of antifungal shampoo twice a week may contribute to reducing the risk of reinfection [2–3].

Viable spores, discovered in fomites such as hairbrushes and combs, emphasize the importance of disinfecting these items for all anthropophilic species. This precaution is particularly crucial for hairstylists, who must ensure the implementation of proper measures to disinfect multiuser equipment. Effective disinfectants, such as bleach or a 2% aqueous solution of sodium hypochlorite containing 16.5% salt, should be used for proper disinfection [4].

There is limited evidence available for the management of asymptomatic carriers of scalp dermatophytosis. It is believed that asymptomatic carriers play an essential role in introducing new infections and sustaining them within communities. Occult disease is often present in over half of family members, including adults. For siblings of individuals with anthropophilic tinea capitis, a thorough examination, including scalp cultures, is recommended to establish their infection status. If the fungal culture results are positive but the scalp appears clinically unaffected, they are categorized as carriers. In such cases, the consensus leans towards using antifungal shampoos for treatment [5]. Topical shampoos containing povidone-iodine or ketoconazole have demonstrated a higher rate of mycological cure (94% and 100%, respectively), making them more effective options for the broader population. Nevertheless, differing opinions persist regarding the appropriate course of action for siblings of children diagnosed with *Trichophyton tonsurans* infection, especially when positive cultures from scalp brushing are present [6].

In individuals with a low conidia load, topical therapies are preferred over systemic treatments. For specific situations, such as persistent asymptomatic carriers or cases with a high conidia load, a combined approach involving oral treatment targeting the involved species alongside topical therapy might be considered. In cases of zoophilic infection, it is crucial to identify and address the animal source. If feasible, it is advisable to clean or wash furniture that regularly comes into direct contact with the affected individual or pet. Analysing culture or molecular identification of the pathogen can offer insights into the probable origin of the infection. Head shaving is considered highly unnecessary [7].

In the event of a tinea outbreak within a household caused by a zoophilic dermatophyte, it is recommended to have the pet, particularly if it was a recent addition, examined by a veterinarian. Additionally, if the patient or other members of the household encounter repeated dermatophyte infections, the animal should undergo a thorough evaluation. Pets might exhibit visible symptoms of dermatophyte infection such as desquamation and hair loss, or they could potentially remain asymptomatic carriers of infection [8].

Moreover, a broader perspective reveals the undeniable impact of social disparities in tinea capitis incidence. A significant study encompassing a large U.S. cohort of Medicaid-insured children demonstrated a stark contrast, with African American children experiencing an incidence rate seven times higher than their White counterparts. Notably, rates of confirmatory diagnostic testing among Medicaid-insured children were notably lower, possibly indicating disparities in care driven by limited resources and time constraints [9]. These findings underscore the pressing need for tailored public health policies and opportunities to bolster outcomes, prevent outbreaks and curtail relapses. In the intricate tapestry of preventive approaches, these insights serve as beacons guiding us towards a more inclusive and effective safeguarding of public health. Future research is needed and should not only address treatment resistance but also monitor changes in epidemiological patterns, social disparities and the emergence of new pathogens.

References

1. Segal E, Elad D. Human and zoonotic dermatophytoses: epidemiological aspects. *Front Microbiol.* 2021;12:713532.
2. Hay RJ. Tinea capitis: current status. *Mycopathologia.* 2017 Feb;182(1–2):87–93.
3. Gupta AK, Mays RR, Versteeg SG, Piraccini BM, Shear NH, Piguet V, Tosti A, Friedlander SF. Tinea capitis in children: a systematic review of management. *J Eur Acad Dermatol Venereol.* 2018 Dec;32(12):2264–74.
4. Fuller LC, Barton RC, Mohd Mustapa MF, Proudfoot LE, Punjabi SP, Higgins EM. British Association of Dermatologists' guidelines for the management of tinea capitis 2014. *Br J Dermatol.* 2014 Sep;171(3):454–63.
5. Aharaz A, Jemec GBE, Hay RJ, Saunte DML. Tinea capitis asymptomatic carriers: what is the evidence behind treatment? *J Eur Acad Dermatol Venereol.* 2021;35(11):2199–207.
6. Bookstaver PB, Watson HJ, Winters SD, Carlson AL, Schulz RM. Prophylactic ketoconazole shampoo for tinea capitis in a high-risk pediatric population. *J Pediatr Pharmacol Ther.* 2011 Jul;16(3):199–203. doi: 10.5863/1551-6776-16.3.199.
7. White JM, Higgins EM, Fuller LC. Screening for asymptomatic carriage of *Trichophyton tonsurans* in household contacts of patients with tinea capitis: results of 209 patients from South London. *J Eur Acad Dermatol Venereol.* 2007;21:1061–4.
8. Kakourou T, Uksal U; European society for pediatric dermatology. Guidelines for the management of tinea capitis in children. *Pediatr Dermatol.* 2010 May–Jun;27(3):226–8.
9. Hennessee IP, Benedict K, Dulski TM, Lipner SR, Gold JAW. Racial disparities, risk factors, and clinical management practices for tinea capitis: an observational cohort study among U.S. children with Medicaid. *J Am Acad Dermatol.* 2023 Aug 5:S0190-9622(23)02418-0.

Index

Note: **Bold** page numbers refer to tables and *italic* page numbers refer to figures.